# YOGA AND INDIAN PHILOSOPHY

KAREL WERNER



MOTILAL BANARSIDASS PUBLISHERS
PRIVATE LIMITED • DELHI

*2nd Corrected Edition: Delhi,* **2017**
*Reprint: Delhi, 1980, 1998*
*First Edition: Delhi, 1977*



ISBN: 978-81-208-0608-5 (Cloth)
ISBN: 978-81-208-1609-1 (Paper)

MOTILAL BANARSIDASS
41 U.A., Bungalow Road, Jawahar Nagar, Delhi 110 007
8 Mahalaxmi Chamber, 22 Bhulabhai Desai Road, Mumbai 400 026
203 Royapettah High Road, Mylapore, Chennai 600 004
236, 9th Main III Block, Jayanagar, Bangalore 560 011
8 Camac Street, Kolkata 700 017
Ashok Rajpath, Patna 800 004
Chowk, Varanasi 221 001

## PREFACE TO THE SECOND EDITION

It is gratifying to see that my first book written in English has been kept in print for so many years, especially when I think of the difficulties I had to get it published in the first place. Although Indian topics were quite popular in the 1970s, my manuscript was not judged popular enough to sell and was rejected by three publishers. One of them expressed the reason succinctly: "It is too highbrow!" Next I offered it to Collins who had been holding the manuscript for a year when I was about to leave for a sabbatical in the autumn of 1975. I wrote a letter complaining about it and received a personal letter of apology from Lady Collins. One referee, Ninian Smart, had been holding the manuscript for a year and it was only after my complaint that he was urged to produce at last his assessment. I was then told that it might take another year or longer to get the book into print if approved.

This was the last straw and I decided to offer it to Banarsidass, publishers from whom I had been frequently buying indological books for myself and the departmental library in Durham. Rather than negotiating by correspondence, I took a copy of the manuscript with me and so it first travelled in my bag around Sri Lanka, then to South India and in a zig zag manner from sea to sea to the north until I reached Delhi in April 1976. On Monday, April 12, I was received by the late Mr. N.P. Jain who was then in charge of the Banarsidass publishing house. In the course of our conversation I mentioned casually my difficulties in getting my book into print. Mr. N.P. Jain immediately said: "Give it to me, I'll get it out in six months and I guarantee that it will never be out of print." The contract was signed on Friday, April 16, 1976, the book was out in January 1977 and the rest is history.

The book, which does not really need any substantial updating and is published with only minor corrections, was recently referred to as a 'classic' by an anonymous reviewer of the proposal for another work of mine. The recommended literature in its first chapter, 'The Existential Situation of Man as Reflected in European and Indian Thought', could be supplemented by titles published subsequently, which are many, but interested readers can easily find information about them in this age 'googling' on line. So it only remains for me to thank the present head of the house, Mr. R.P. Jain, for honouring the promise of his late brother to keep the book in print.

Karel Werner

London, 24 October 2014.

## CONTENTS

## A NOTE ON PRONUNCIATION AND TRANSLITERATION

Sanskrit vowels are pronounced as in Italian or in Czech: *a* as in English *shut*, *i* as in *pit*, *u* as in *bull*; *e* and *o* were originally diphthongs and are pronounced long, as in *fair* and *cause*, respectively. Real diphthongs *ai* and *au* are pronounced so as to make both constituents of the diphthong audible. *Ṛ* is considered to be a vowel and has the function of one. It is pronounced as in Czech *brk*. New Indian pronunciation is *ri* as in *river* and this is often used in transliteration (*rig*, *Sanskrit* instead of *ṛg*, *Sanskṛt*). *Ā*, *ī*, *ū* are long vowels.

Consonants are pronounced almost as in English. Diacritical marks in the form of dots under (*ṭ*) or above (*ṅ*) them can be ignored (except in *ṣ*). *C* is pronounced as *ch* in English *chin*. *Ñ* is pronounced soft as in Spanish *mañana* (the same sound as *ny* in the Russian name *Vanya*). *H* following a consonant is always pronounced, including after *t* and *d*, so that *th* sounds like *t* and *h* in *pothole*, *dh* like in *godhead*, *ch* like in *beachhead*. Both *ś* and *ṣ* can be pronounced as *sh*, although there is a slight difference in Indian pronunciation.

There are no generally observed rules of transliteration of Indian names. Current transliteration of names known from various publications and belonging to famous personalities has been retained without using diacritical marks (e.g. Ramakrishna, the modern saint). Names of historical or mythological figures have been given in their correct form (e.g. Rāma and Kṛṣṇa, the two incarnations of Viṣṇu). Differing spellings in titles of books quoted have been preserved.

# LIST OF ABBREVIATIONS

| | |
|---|---|
| Ait. Br. | Aitareya Brāhmaṇa |
| Ait. Up. | Aitareya Upaniṣad |
| AN | Aṅguttara Nikāya |
| AV | Atharva Veda |
| Bṛh. Up. | Bṛhadāraṇyaka Upaniṣad |
| Chānd. Up. | Chāndogya Upaniṣad |
| DN | Dīgha Nikāya |
| Kauṣ.Up. | Kauṣītaki Brāhmaṇa Upaniṣad |
| Maitrī Up. | Maitrī or Maitrāyaṇīya Upaniṣad |
| Māṇḍ. Up. | Māṇḍūkya Upaniṣad |
| MN | Majjhima Nikāya |
| PTS | Pāli Text Society |
| RV | Ṛg Veda |
| Sam. N. | Saṁyutta Nikāya |
| SBE | Sacred Books of the East |
| SN | Sutta Nipāta |
| Śat. Br. | Śatapatha Brāhmaṇa |
| Śvet. Up. | Śvetāśvatara Upaniṣad |
| Tait. Br. | Taittirīya Brāhmaṇa |
| Tait. Up. | Taittirīya Upaniṣad |

# INTRODUCTION

Much has already been written on Indian philosophy, and still more on Yoga. While the themes falling within the confines of Indian philosophy have been dealt with predominantly in voluminous works or the expert papers of scholars specialised in the subject, Yoga has become notorious as a rewarding topic for writers of popular books which make hardly any attempt at a historical and comprehensive survey of it.

It is not surprising that Indian philosophy has been neglected by our popular literature. There has never been close communication in the West between academic philosophers and historians of philosophy on the one hand and the general public on the other. And philosophy itself has never become an attraction for the masses, regrettable though that may be. Furthermore, if Indian philosophy is treated with our Western conceptual equipment and our traditional academic approach to the history of human thought, its character is inevitably changed or a picture of it is given which fails to reveal its essence. And that deprives it of its chief allure.[1]

Indian philosophy, on the other hand, has never been purely academic. It has always preserved its vital links with the situation of man and its interest in the place that he may occupy in the universe. Besides, it has not dealt with man's situation only in general, but has been concerned with it from the standpoint of the individual. In other words, it has been predominantly or to a great extent *existential*. This feature, although admitted by most modern historians of Indian philosophy, naturally gets overlooked in the course of giving conceptual accounts of the schools of Indian thought.

1. This has been done not only by Western scholars like Paul Deussen, in his *Allgemeine Geschichte der Philosophie*, vol. 1, 1-3—who based his work chiefly on textual criticism, but also by Indian authors who received European education, such as S. Radhakrishnan—*Indian Philosophy*, vols. I-II, or S. Dasgupta—*A History of Indian Philosophy*, vols. I-V. Both these scholars have adopted the Western academic method of description of Indian ideas and consequently their works have never become widely read.

Yet it is important to realise that, as far as the creators of Indian philosophical teachings were concerned, philosophy was a matter of life and death, in the same way as, or perhaps even more than, it was for Socrates in ancient Greece. Philosophy in ancient India was, above all, a practical quest for truth or atleast for guidelines pointing to truth, and the practical application of those guidelines was paramount. Conceptual elaboration and systemisation came second.

Indian philosophy has preserved its special character, particularly its closeness to man's life and its concern for his destiny, mainly owing to its relation to Yoga. It is true that it was affected and stimulated also by various other elements, quite often by disputations and arguments with religious doctrines, and this can be said about philosophy in Europe as well. But from the time of the Upaniṣads—or even earlier—till Aurobindo it has been Yoga which has provided an important source of inspiration for Indian philosophical thought.

Its link with Yoga is no doubt the chief appeal of Indian philosophy for laymen in the West and it is also the reason for the reputation it has acquired among them without its being really known. Stemming perhaps from the lack of comprehensive and readable treatises on Indian philosophical teachings which would pay proper regard to their relation to Yoga, it has become the habit of popular writers on Yoga to convey some distorted bits of Indian philosophical teachings to their readers as a kind of "Yoga philosophy". Both terms, Yoga and philosophy, have therefore become confused and it seems impossible to draw a distinct line between them. In academic histories of Indian philosophy Yoga is seldom considered to be anything more than one of the six orthodox systems of philosophy indiscernible, in its metaphysical conclusions, from the Sāṅkhya system. Yet in reality Yoga in one form or another plays an important or at least a recognised part in all the six systems as well as in Buddhism, Jainism and even in the thought of the time prior to the appearance of all these doctrines.

When dealing with philosophy and Yoga we have therefore to distinguish between them, while at the same time pointing out their mutual relation, which is often that of interdependence. This is, of course, no easy task, since even nowadays philosophers find it difficult to explain what philosophy actually is and nobody has so far attempted to give a clear definition of Yoga for the purpose of philosophical enquiry.[1] But broadly speaking we may regard philosophy as a constant endeavour of the human mind to describe and rationally explain experienced reality in clearly defined concepts and create an overall and systematic as well as intuitively penetrative picture of the world including man which satisfies man's intellectual curiosity or urge for formulated knowledge.

Yoga, on the other hand, is always a practical activity on the part of the whole individual. It appears to be a consciously adopted system of training or pattern of behaviour aiming at enlarging or deepening man's direct experience of reality rather than his ability to describe and explain it.

This being so, we can see that philosophy appears at work wherever a Yogi tries to describe and explain his experiences, but it has also already appeared before he became a Yogi, because taking up the practice of Yoga is always preceded by a certain motivation which may certainly itself be looked upon as a rudimentary or initial philosophical view which is to be clarified, enhanced or modified by new experience gained through Yoga.

This is why it may be a worthwhile undertaking to write about Indian philosophy and Yoga in one book while trying to distinguish the one from the other, and to show the different degrees of their relatedness, interdependence and antagonism at various times and in various schools.

The fact that Indian philosophy is predominantly existential and that the starting point of Yoga activities is the individual's awareness of the situation in which he finds himself provides us with the opportunity to compare the European existential analysis of the human situation with the Indian view, and to point out the basic similarities in the structure of life as it is experienced by the individual in different times and cultures.

1. Some scholars writing on Indian religious and philosophical thought are aware of the problem involved in dealing with Yoga and do give useful hints and views about its nature. So, E. Conze in *Buddhist Thought in India*, London 1962, pp. 17-21. But the question of the nature of Yoga and its relation to philosophy and religion would certainly merit a separate and more thorough analysis than could be afforded in this book.

The subject of the first chapter is thus a natural start to the book.

The book is based on material which has been used by the author in academic courses as well as in classes of adult education. It is by no means an exhaustive study of the two topics —Yoga and Indian philosophy—and their mutual relation. All it can hope to achieve is to provide a framework for further study and, perhaps, a stimulus for more research. It is intended to be read by those members of the general public who are interested in the theme and therefore it has been made as readable as possible, while at the same time preserving its standard as a reliable introduction to Indian philosophical teachings and the teachings of Yoga for a student of the subjects. One or two points in it might be accepted, it is hoped, as original contributions to research within the field of the theme. And, finally, the author could hardly avoid having his own reflections on some of the issues dealt with, which are highly relevant to everybody's life and therefore deserve to be treated not only objectively, but also with some portion of personal involvement.

Chapter I

# THE EXISTENTIAL SITUATION OF MAN AS REFLECTED IN EUROPEAN AND INDIAN THOUGHT

Western philosophy for a long time did not concern itself genuinely with the existential situation of the individual. Philosophical thought is noted for its generalised approach in dealing with reality, including man, and although the concept of man is based, in the first instance, on our having an individual and direct experience of being individual men (in spite of the fact that we share certain qualities that make us all alike), concern for the individual seems to have been banned from the mainstream of philosophy for reasons never properly stated.

It may now seem natural to us that what can properly be called philosophical thinking started in ancient Greece with reflections on the nature of the world or universe and that the desideratum of the first philosophers was to find out the substance underlying the world. But it seems natural to us only because the whole of our civilisation is the result of the extraverted attitude of the Western mind with its eagerness to conquer nature and her resources. Man himself thus comes to be regarded as a mere accidental product of the various processes going on in nature, and his mental life with all its emotions, rational thought, aesthetic and other values is regarded as only a by-product of chemical and electrical reactions in his nervous system.

It is of course true that already at the dawn of Greek history the Greek mind was preoccupied with men and important questions concerning his individual destiny and his relation to the supernatural and the Divine, as revealed in the teaching of the Orphics. But that was a period in which thinking about these problems had still not developed the capacity for abstraction, was purely religious and expressed its ideas in mythological language. It is only with the Milesian school that the history of Western philosophy begins and here is found the start of extraverted investigation of the world, when the activity of the human mind turned in a direction that finally led to the birth of science and its domination over our lives and thought.

This shows that the objectivistic method of inquiry into reality was felt to be unsatisfactory, which opened a possibility of investigating the problems of human existence from the individual's point of view. In fact, already at an early stage there had occurred in Greek philosophical development a revolt against the onesided objectivistic approach to reality which disregarded that quality of mental life manifested in the human personality which is capable of moral judgments and actions. This was the movement of sophists who finally arrived at the dictum that man was the measure of all things (Protagoras). But it seems that the sophists were pragmatists in the sense that they were interested in the business of everday life rather than in metaphysical problems concerning the individual and his destiny. They seem to have been sceptics as well. Nevertheless one might assume that an inquiry into the status of the individual not only within society, but also in the world at large and in life in general, would have been possible. But the trend was diverted elsewhere because of Socrates, the man who is still much of a mystery for the historians of ancient Greek philosophy, and who can be looked upon as the peak in the development of Sophism while at the same time representing a new beginning of objective inquiry into the nature of reality as grasped by the human mind. He was not worried by the problem of a first principle or the nature of the world but was concerned about the values experienced by a man in his life, such as what is good and what is evil, what is beauty, virtue, duty, what is right and wrong, and how some form of certainty and general consent may be reached about them. But in dealing with these relative values and the way they were understood by people, Socrates seems to have ascribed to them some form of objective and independent nature and he aimed at exact definitions which would be valid in every situation and for every man.

As a result of this quest for objectivity of values, which in fact only exist when experienced by individual subjects, the experiencing individual was, in the long run, finally lost sight of—and he is still missing in the structure of our scientifically oriented, objectivistic civilisation. In philosophy, however, this experiencing individual *has* recently been rediscovered—by the modern existentialists—and acknowledged as the most important factor of reality, although, and this is significant, the impetus came from the sphere of religious thinking, from Kierkegaard a man who was seriously worried by the fate and destiny of the individual.

Why it took so long for philosophy to start to be interested in the individual and his existential situation and why this interest has never become general in modern Western philosophy—and is even looked down upon by many specialists in non-metaphysical fields of philosophical research work—can only be explained by the force and strength of the foundations laid for our Western civilisation by ancient Greek thought. It may, in a simplified way, be best summarised by referring to the two most outstanding continuators of Socratic philosophy, namely Plato and Aristotle.

Plato continued Socrates' preoccupation with general ideas and considered that those with ethical and aesthetic significance were the highest in the order of reality. He pushed further their supposed objectivity in postulating their independent metaphysical existence in the world of ideas of which our world of things and human experience is only a faint reflection or shadow. This Platonic idealism has had a profound influence on European thinking—in medieval times through the teachings of the Church—and is probably still responsible for the fact that ideas and ideologies are, even in our secularised and materialistic era, more powerful and decisive than realistic conclusions based on existential analysis of the concrete situation.

Aristotle, although he criticised and rejected Plato's theory of ideas, continued Socrates' trend in his doctrine of universals in which he introduced new concepts, such as substance and essence, and defined concepts of form and matter in a new way. On the whole his metaphysic is not altogether clear, but he made a vast step beyond the mere attempt of Socrates at clear definitions in creating a whole system of logic. In this respect he further strengthened the objectivistic tendency in philosophy and at the same time laid the foundations for later scientific development.

It is true that after Aristotle we find one or two schools of ancient philosophy which—like that of the sophists—were centred around man, but they did not exercise much influence on the trend towards objectivistic thinking and themselves were dependent on contemporary prescientific theories when they described the world. The most important of them was Stoicism. The Stoics—following Socrates in that respect—were greatly preoccupied with ethics. They genuinely tried, above all, to solve the question of human freedom in a world governed, as they believed, by cosmic determinism. They found themselves to be under the pressure of circumstances and events beyond their control, so they resorted to emphasizing the control of their own minds in maintaining calm and virtue under all conditions. In the context of their cosmic philosophy, however, man as an individual has little chance, if any, to gain some command over his destiny. Their abstract ideal of a perfect wise man seemed even to them beyond man's capacity and so there was little more to be done in practical life beyond compromising with what life brought or else committing suicide when compromise was impossible or too humiliating.

Although the ethical teachings of Stoicism were of a very high standard, they were not backed by an adequate explanation of the individual's place in the scheme of the cosmos with its rule of necessity. Therefore their ethics required religious grounds for their justification. It is not surprising that Christianity adopted much of the Stoics' ethical doctrine.

In Christianity the living problems of the individual and his destiny were thoroughly externalised and petrified by a system of dogmas into a rigid doctrine. The concern for the individual in all forms of Christian philosophy derived from his supposed destiny after death as laid down in that doctrine, and the significance of his actual existential situation and his own experience of himself and his destiny was not seen (with the exception of a few mystics). All that was needed was faith in the doctrine and conformity to the prescribed code of religious behaviour.

The first philosopher to question the established way of philosophising was Descartes, who thus started modern philosophy. He wanted to have a firmer basis for philosophy than mere faith. He was, in fact, already a modern scientist and felt that philosophy should be a science which consequently should be based on firm empirical knowledge (knowledge, of course, which had to be "objective", i.e. verifiable by external evidence, accessible to everyone). In this he created a problem for philosophy which, in our century, almost killed it.

Descartes' requirement cannot be met by philosophy and is entirely unjustified. It would mean transforming philosophy into a science or making it into a kind of science above sciences. But philosophy cannot become a science among other sciences, because it has no specialised object or separate field of inquiry of its own; it has been and still is concerned with the nature of the whole of reality. On this basis the claim could be, and indeed was, made of philosophy being the Queen of sciences. But this also is an untenable proposition, not only because scientists would never accept it, but also because each science itself does the work philosophy would be expected to do for it, in forming scientific theories and working hypotheses. For these reasons it was thought that philosophy, in the age of science, was no more possible or, at any rate, certainly not necessary. However, philosophy has survived and has shown in recent times an enormous vitality. When the present trend to limit it to the field of linguistic analysis and the history of human thought wears itself out, this vitality may again bring it into the forefront in a world troubled by problems that have been created as by-products of science.

The heart of the problem may lie in the fact that philosophy, although always trying to be objective and universal, nevertheless cannot at any given moment be anything else than a reflection of reality as experienced, understood and interpreted by a philosophising individual in a certain existential situation, no matter how hard he tries to abstract himself from his situation or, for that matter, from the fact that he is an individual and a man, not an abstract subject or impersonal mind-machine.

Descartes certainly started rightly by doubting everything, including the fact of his own existence. In other words he not only did not want to take anything for granted, but he did not even want to rely on any second-hand evidence. That was at least his starting position and if he had persevered with it, he would have brought philosophy much further than he did.

The first fact which Descartes established for himself as certain was his own existence. He based this certainty on the experience of thinking. Doubting is also a form of thinking and so if there is a process of doubting going on, there must inevitably be someone who is doing the doubting and this someone is I. "I think, therefore I am" is the famous dictum of

Descartes. But this is about his only contribution to existential philosophy. And significantly enough, he did not thus establish for himself the fact of his own existence through a direct act of being aware of self-existence, but through reasoning, i. e. through the indirect process of a logical conclusion, as if the self-awareness or the experience of self-existence were not possible without, or did not precede, the process of thinking.

Starting with the laboriously established fact of his own existence Descartes proceeded only too quickly to establish the whole known world around us, not really by following his own method of "clear and distinct perception", but again through reasoning based on indirect evidence, mostly relying on the existence of God for which he used an old scholastic proof.

Thus at the beginning of the modern period in European philosophy the objectivistic channel of philosophising appears to have been so deeply ingrained in the minds of philosophers that even the doubting Descartes was eager to outline a picture of an impersonal world in which man himself figures as a very unimportant entity—in fact already as unimportant as an individual person is in our present technical civilisation and in totalitarian political systems. For this Descartes and subsequent philosophers may be blamed. For Descartes came very close to the starting-point of a real existential analysis without elaborating it or making use of the opportunity and, regrettably, it was not even taken up by any of the subsequent philosophers who, instead, elaborated on Descartes' theories of the material world or of the immaterial mind, doing so always in an objectifying or even absolutising way. Hegel seems to have been the culmination of this trend at one extreme and Marxist philosophy at the other. In Hegel it is Spirit that underlies the evolution of the world, in Marxism it is matter—in both cases we have an abstract concept which does not in the least help man to understand himself and his situation. When abstractions substitute entirely for the actual experience and concrete knowledge of the individual in philosophy, political and economic theory finds it easy to disregard the individual, his rights and even his existence.

In this way philosophy, which had freed itself from domination by impersonal religious doctrine, failed to free man from domination by impersonal abstract conceptions. Religion promised man salvation if he gave up his individuality and freedom of inquiry into his status and destiny. Political theories based on dogmatic philosophy mostly inspired by Hegelian absolutism promised man temporary salvation on earth—practically for the same price.

A protest against the inadequacy of modern philosophical thought as well as the religious insufficiency of Protestantism, which maintained an impersonal dogmatism not very different from that of Roman Christianity, came at last from a philosopher who was deeply religiously committed. He was S. Kierkegaard (1813-55), whose philosophy stemmed from his concern for truth, truth that he as an individual faced in the crucial moment of choice whether to believe or not. In his youth an ardent student of Hegel, he was soon disappointed by Hegel's speculative philosophy. He then refused all the usual objective criteria of truth whether based on scientific evidence or on the rationalised dogmas of the religious establishment. The truth for him was personal and could be acquired only by a painful process of appropriating it. This could be done only by way of an absolutely binding decision to believe in God. This decision was absolute because it was taken in complete isolation and the individual was totally responsible for it. The result of this choice was an experience of "passionate inwardness" which, however, did not resolve the problem once and for all. Although there was growth of the sense of inwardness, the agony did not diminish. The decision to believe had to be taken time and again. If it was not being renewed inwardly and absolutely over and over again, it was not valid.

Most of what Kierkegaard wrote is in its content hardly notable in our time. What has, however, remained influential in modern existential philosophy and is humanly highly relevant is his consistent attitude of total ethical responsibility for truth in an individual's life, which is the result of his choice. In this way the point was again made, for the first time since Socrates, that philosophy is a personal quest for truth with implications for the individual person's way of life and not just an objective inquiry into the nature of the world around.

Insofar as this point is incorporated in existentialism it can claim, as Sartre did for it, that it is a "humanism", i. e. a philosophy whose point of gravity lies in human personal life rather than in non-human ("inhuman", "alienated") objective reality. At the same time, however, scientific progress introduced into philosophy the method of analysis which was, for philosophy, particularly elaborated by phenomenologists. Modern existentialists have applied phenomenological analysis to the human situation with considerable success.

These two elements—the "humanism" of their philosophy and the method of phenomenological analysis—enabled modern existentialists to make some discoveries for Western philosophy which are well worth noting (even though some of them are not actual discoveries, but the introduction into philosophy of an accurate conceptual formulation of man's everyday psychological experience).

The first of these discoveries is the uniqueness of individual human existence, which can never be externalised or universalised as, for example, the existence of a television set or a mathematical formula can. Although man forms a concept of humanity or mankind, this concept can never have any kind of objective content, but is only an expansion of every man's concrete subjective awareness of existing as a particular human being among others. The actual conscious existence of the individual always remains the basis and indispensable condition for any kind of philosophy, not only for the philosophy of existence, including the philosophy of "Existence", but also, for that matter, for any branch of science, even if proper account of this fact is seldom taken in them.

Secondly comes the recognition that conscious human existence always involves an awareness of the "world". Man or consciousness never exist on their own, but a man or a consciousness always finds him- or itself (=himself or itself) in some environment, i.e. in the world. "Being-in-the-world" is therefore the basic structure of human existence or, obviously, of any concrete existence, while "existence as such" or any general idea of existence exists as an abstract concept only as long as there is at least one individual consciousness capable of conceiving such an idea. If, however, Existence or Being in general is asserted, as was done among existentialists by

Heidegger, it is no longer a product of phenomenological analysis, but rather a metaphysical postulate.

The third point concerns a somewhat complicated problem which could in itself be the subject of an historical inquiry ranging from ancient to modern times. It is expressed by the existential dictum that existence is prior to essence. In simple terms it means that there is no definite structure of man prior to his existence (in the sense of a Platonic idea of "manhood" or of an Aristotelian substance of what makes man a man), but rather that in existing every man constantly creates his manhood and its particular expression, the different modifications of his nature. The structure of human existence lies in its ceaseless sequence of subjective confrontations of the individual with the fact of existing, which implies choosing to live (or not to live) in a certain way; and just that is the recurrent act forming man's essence, which thus undergoes constant modifications throughout his life.

When analysing further the basic structure of human existence, as man experiences it, the existentialists arrived at three other important elements of their philosophy: that of despair, that of death and that of freedom.

The source of despair is man's being thrown upon himself with respect to choosing the course his actions should follow in the absence on the one hand of the spontaneity of animal instincts, and on the other of any firm religious belief. On self-reflection man realises that he is alone in the world, facing inescapable limitations like death, suffering, conflict and liability to error, while being absolutely responsible for choosing his own course of actions by which he determines for himself his essence.

Death is a fact of human existence which seems accidental and absurd to Sartre, depriving life of all its obvious meaning. It posits an apparent limit to man's existence as he knows it from his experience, i. e. to his 'being-in-the-world', without any promise or hope. There seems to be no remedy for it, therefore it has to be accepted. For Heidegger it represents one of man's personal possibilities which is supreme among them as it allows him to extinguish them all. But whether chosen, accepted as it comes or banished from man's consciousness, death is the essential constituent of the structure of personal existence and no philosophical system which ignores it can claim to have taken into account all the important elements of reality.

Freedom and being aware of the fact of being free is as inescapable a part of the structure of man's existence as birth or death. Despite all the external limitations he faces in every situation, man is condemned to be free internally all the time, even if he tries to hide it from himself behind a (chosen) adherence to an external authority. He has to choose the course of his external actions and bear the responsibility inasmuch as he thereby determines his essence, i.e. shapes his character and his status, and constitutes himself on the level of being himself. Freedom in the existentialist sense is not a property of human nature but is human existence, which is not "a form of being, but a form of doing, of choosing and making itself".[1]

When philosophy is concerned with these fundamental aspects of human existence, it is far from being made superfluous by science, because these aspects are entirely beyond the capacity of science, yet vital to man as problems to be faced, worked upon and thought about, religion having lost its power to persuade man that it has solved them for him. As long as man ignores these vital constituents of his existence, he lives a spurious sort of life which the existentialists call "inauthentic". This is so whether he ignores them because of negligence or because he has accepted the "objectified" explanation of his existence given by science or because he believes in and follows the authoritatively formulated teaching of an established religious system. In each of these cases man, in fact, chooses an "inauthentic" existence, refusing to live fully to his human capacity, which demands from him a full intellectual grasping of both his human situation in general and every single situation he faces in particular; a fully conscious decision to live (or not to live) his life, as well as decisions taken repeatedly in every concrete circumstance; and, finally, full acceptance of responsibility for his life and all decisions made by him.

As being free is an aspect of being a man, the attempt to ignore this fact is again, basically, the free choice of an inauthentic form of existence which does not enable a man to es-

1. H.J. Blackham, *Six Existentialist Thinkers*, London 1956, p. 129.

cape from full personal responsibility for it. To face consciously the facts of one's existence with the implied necessity to choose its direction and, to some extent, its contents ("to form one's essence") means to lead a real life which the existentialists designate as "authentic".

The most urgent call to authentic existence comes from the inevitable fact of death. In inauthentic existence man covers his sense of insecurity and frustration in face of the inevitability of death by falsely objectifying it as a phenomenon common to all and not particular to him. In this way he may temporarily remove the fact of his personal death from the focus of his attention and achieve a false sense of balance and safety, but he thus loses the only firm value of his life—the chance to live authentically. If man faces the fact of his personal death and lives in constant awareness of it, anticipating its possibility any moment, he becomes singularly awake to the significance of every decision and choice that he makes and his life takes the course of a fully conscious and self-responsible authentic existence.

With some existentialists this idea of authentic existence points to some form of transcendence which is anticipated by man at least as a possibility (Jaspers). It is indicated that it may become a personal experience which, however, is not to be made into an object of impersonal inquiry. For existentialists of all shades truth remains personal and cannot be objectified. This was already the case with Kierkegaard who revolted against the Hegelian conceptual description of being, as well as against the pursuit of "the objective way" of approaching God, which is entirely impossible, "because God is a subject and therefore exists only for subjectivity in inwardness"[1] and "is never a third party when he is present in the religious consciousness; this is precisely the secret of the religious consciousness."[2] Hence also his refusal of any formulated church doctrine and establishment. And that also is why Jaspers does not want to attempt to describe transcendence. He admits, however, that one can "bear witness" to it. And that certainly has implications: a witness to transcendence must undoubtedly have an

1. *Concluding Unscientific Postscript* p. 178, quoted by Blackham, *op. cit.*, p. 20

2. *Concluding Unscientific Postscript* p. 61; Blackham, p. 20.

inner experience to live by, a personal direct source of strength which does not need theoretical formulation and objective justification. In this way existentialism leads to recognition of transcendence and of the possibility of experiencing it.

Materialist existentialists, like Sartre, although profoundly interested in awakening the feeling of authentic existence when they are experiencing the "dread" in the face of "being thrown" into a responsibility for themselves as well as for "the whole world", ignore the finger pointing the way out of this thinker's riddle into the anticipation of the experience of transcendence which Jaspers or even Heidegger seem to have found a consistent further step when they had reached the utmost peak conceptual thought can climb. Nevertheless the consistency of that step is, indirectly, proved even by Sartre. It is not possible to remain true to one's philosophy when it is purely conceptual and brings one into a thinker's cul-de-sac. If the step towards the individual encounter with transcendence is not taken, there must either be a return to or acceptance of religious faith (as in the case of Gabriel Marcel) or else the thinker embraces an external doctrine that reduces for him the dread stemming from the responsibility he feels for the peopled world and that shows him the direction for action—whether in social reforms or in revolution.

In both cases it is an escape from the full responsibility of a thinker and philosopher and is virtually the choice of the inauthentic form of life. In Sartre's case the philosophical fiasco is remarkable. He has found the lacking direction for his action (which his limited existentialist outlook does not give him) in Marxism. But from the existentialist standpoint Marxism cannot but be classified as an arrogant dogmatism which not only imposes external discipline in action, but controls thinking as well, aiming thereby at abolishing the freedom of the individual and offering him the transfer of the burden of his individual responsibility to the collective, which is virtually impossible. Hence Sartre's oscillation and wavering.

So it seems quite natural and logical for consistent existentialism to point or lead, in the last instance, to the threshold of transcendence and then to leave it to the individual to work out for himself any further conclusions and steps. And as we have already indicated, this is so even with Heidegger. He was careful to set himself the task merely of exploring the structure of being within strictly conceptual boundaries of philosophy. In the course of his analysis, however, he used the description of personal existence[1] in order to elucidate the concept of the transcendent Being-in-itself. To postulate such a concept in this way implies personal acceptance of its reality, and if that is not based on faith, either religious or metaphysical, the possibility of experiencing it has to be admitted or indicated, for it certainly cannot be proved on rational grounds. In his later writings Heidegger indeed indicated that the transcendent Being-in-itself could become accessible to experience, although he never produced a full answer to the problem and his chief work has remained unfinished.[2]

* * *

1. Which he, of course, could not avoid when using the method of phenomenological analysis which was designed for the study of the concrete, experienced consciousness.

2. Literature on existentialism is vast. Most works of existentialist thinkers are already available in English translation. As an introduction for the general public the following book is of interest, as it deals also with phenomenology: Colin Wilson : *Introduction to the New Existentialism*, London, 1966.

Besides the book by Blackham, the following books may be recommended : E.L. Allen; *Existentialism from Within*, London, 1953; W. Desen : *The Tragic Finale. An Essay on the Philosophy of Jean-Paul Sartre*, Cambridge 1954; F. H. Heinmann : *Existentialism and the Modern Predicament*, 2nd edition, London, 1954.

For a comparison of existentialist philosophy with Indian ways of thinking the following works may be studied : Guru Dutt : *Existentialism and Indian Thought*. 3rd edition, Bangalore, 1960; G. Srinivasan : *The Existentialist Concepts and the Hindu Philosophical Systems*, Allahabad, 1967.

It may not appear very prudent to try to gain recognition for Indian philosophy—and for Yoga—by showing its affinity with some findings of modern European Existentialism for the same reason for which Professor John Passmore apologises for dealing with existentialism at all, for "it lies on the periphery of British philosophical consciousness; it stands, to British philosophers, for continental excess and rankness." (But he adds in a footnote : "In the US, however, existentialism and phenomenology are steadily growing in respectability, although they are often interpreted 'in the spirit of William James'." See his book *A Hundred Years of Philosophy*, London, 1966, p. 176, first published 1957.)

However, existential philosophy as understood in this book has a

Unlike in Europe, philosophy in India has always been concerned with the individual, his existential situation, his destiny and salvation, i.e. with the final solution of the riddle of man's existence. The world or the universe—although the question of its origin is the theme of one of the earliest Indian philosophical texts (the hymn of Creation, RV. 10, 129)—soon appears to be viewed mainly as the stage on which the drama of life is going on. The important and central problem of philosophical investigation is the nature of man and the means of transcending his present limited situation.

This does not mean that Indian philosophy has not been preoccupied with speculations on the nature of the world, even in great detail, but it has never really looked at the world as an objective reality entirely independent of what we call the perceiving subject or as originally utterly devoid of the element of consciousness or mentality (with the exception of the early materialist school known only from fragmentary allusions to it in secondary sources). Nor does it mean that Indian philosophy did not develop specialised disciplines like the theory of knowledge or logic. But even in them the driving force was usually the concern for man and his final destiny: Nāgārjuna, for example, developed his dialectical logic with the intention of showing that final truth could not be found and formulated by logic and lay therefore beyond the grasp of the intellect and could be achieved by direct experience only.

Apart from the fact that Indian philosophy has not fallen into the extreme of totally objectifying reality and divorcing it from the only real source of knowing it, i.e., from intelligent consciousness, there has been another advantage in the develop-

wider significance than the modern European existentialism. The main point to be stressed is that every true philosophy has to be concerned with existence in general and man's existence and its meaning in particular. The post-war European existentialism has to be credited with having made this point again in a time when philosophy was divorced from life and was split into several specialised academic disciplines without a specific task of its own. Even the "British philosophical consciousness" will sooner or later take this point.

ment of Indian thought, namely this, that philosophy has never become subservient to religious dogma, and religious thought has never ignored the results of philosophical investigation. Indian philosophy did not become existential after a failure of religion to satisfy man's urge to be given or shown solutions of the problems of human life and destiny in a way acceptable to his intelligence—as happened in the West. Philosophy and religion in India have mostly been developing side by side, often in some form of collaboration and often influencing each other. What has been highly conceptually formulated in philosophical texts has been, in a more popular way, expressed in religious symbolism, mythical tales and ceremonial rites and vice versa. Although, of course, there also were periods of antagonism and polemics.

The third and most important point in the development of the Indian mind, keeping it in touch with actual human experience, is the part played by Yoga. Yoga as a practical discipline, a method used individually but accepted universally, has always been used in India on the one hand as a means of confirming or testing the results of philosophical investigation and speculation on transcendence and on the other as a source of inspiration and a stimulus for philosophical thinking. Simultaneously Yoga has been adopted by religion as a way of approach to the transcendent, represented by the religious mind in the form of various figures and images of the Divine, and it has been modified by religion to suit the devotional aspect of the human heart (Bhakti Yoga). And further, it was as early as at the beginning of systematic philosophical thought in India that the Buddha proclaimed his direct way of penetrating to the knowledge of truth (in other words, his method of Yoga leading to the experience of the transcendent) to be independent of and above religious teachings as well as philosophical speculation.

In this situation philosophy often became a bridge between following some form of traditional religious practice and the radical adoption of a full Yoga practice. For the individual who had become aware of the inadequacy of the traditional religious outlook based on mere faith, philosophy was able to clarify his existential situation and point out to him the direction in which he could apply his personal effort in search of a direct solution.

Preoccupied as it was with man's existential situation almost from the start, Indian philosophy did not develop that sharp division between the individual and the world[1] which results for the individual in a feeling of complete alienation from the world he sees himself as having been "thrown" into without ever having had any influence on the matter, which is how the basic situation appears to most European existentialists. The basic situation of man in Indian philosophy—as a starting-point for a philosophical inquiry or existential analysis—is rather the elementary fact of man's existence, namely that man is enclosed in his own stream of conscious experience. This view implies that man is not faced with a hostile or indifferent world of solid matter and objective processes going on in an unconscious reality around him, but that he is confronted with processes going on in his own consciousness which have to be analysed and understood in order to get to know his exact existential situation.

This is obviously a phenomenological approach which had been adopted by some Indian systems long before phenomenology came into existence in Europe. As we have seen: when Descartes sought a firm starting-point for his philosophy whose existence would be beyond doubt, he returned to himself as a thinking subject. The direct experience of the thinking process guaranteed, for him, the existence of one who was thinking. However, this is not a phenomenological approach, but a speculative conclusion. The phenomenon of thinking cannot, unfortunately, prove the ultimate existence of a thinking subject, of the individual. This has been shown by Descartes' followers: Descartes proceeded hastily from his first conclusion to the estab-

1. With the exception of the Sāṅkhya system where in theory the *puruṣa*, the individual Self or Spirit, is completely independent of the world and takes no active part in its processes. The empirical personality is entirely the product of the processes going on in nature (*prakṛti*) and the *puruṣa* sees himself being involved in them only by mistake. From the point of view of phenomenological analysis, however, the important part to deal with would be just the empirical personality and the existential situation it finds itself in, *puruṣa* being a metaphysical postulate.

lishment of the firm existence of the world around us, but others after him followed the idealistic suggestion contained in his argument and drew further metaphysical conclusions from it, developing systems of idealist metaphysics which in the end entirely lost sight of and regard for the individual who stood at the beginning of it all; and those who stuck to the individual subject and followed this line of Descartes' argument ended, logically, in the deadlock of solipsism.

Indian philosophy has been saved from these dead ends by its recognition of the conditionality of existence, not only of the experienced world but also of the experiencing subject. It does not absolutise either of them, but its metaphysical schools rather postulate an impersonal and immaterial principle[1] and try to find the ways in which both the individual and the world are related or linked to it. This is the speculative and conceptual approach to the crucial problem of existence. In their practical approach to the solution of the existential problem, which is generally missing in European philosophical endeavours but was present in some form in ancient schools such as that of Pythagoras and is alluded to by some existentialists like Jaspers without being elaborated, the Indian systems usually adopt the empirical method of studying consciousness in an impersonal way both in its inner structure and in its relation to the external world, and they try to deepen the experience by special mental practices involving a training in self-observation and in mind-control which is mostly referred to as Yoga. The practice of self-observation may be compared with the modern phenomenological method of studying consciousness as it functions, while the practice of mind-control is a specific Yoga discipline comparable only to a minor degree with some trends in modern psychology in psycho-analytical schools.

Indian philosophy can also claim to possess the feature of humanism, since man's position in it is central. Man, not the world, is the starting point of philosophical inquiry and although the final solution is envisaged in transcendence, it is, in the Indian view, the human mind which is the only instrument capable of grasping the significance of this term and of

1. *Brahman, Ātman, Puruṣa, Nirvāṇa, Śūnyatā.*

preparing itself for a direct experience of whatever transcendence may really be.

In view of what has been said it will be understood that the points which in Western philosophy have been raised only recently by existentialism have in Indian philosophy always been a legitimate concern for inquiry. The uniqueness of individual human existence is stressed in all systems and confirmed by references to the strictly individual Yoga practice which should enable the individual, on the application of his own effort, to transcend the limitations of his individuality. The recognition that conscious human experience always involves an awareness of the world so that being a man implies "being-in-the-world" is expressed in the Indian concept of Saṃsāra which can be broadly interpreted as "being caught in the world process of becoming". Some systems, like Buddhism, describe consciousness as never existing on its own but always as being conscious of something. Systems which do maintain the concept of "pure consciousness" describe it as a kind of transcendental reality which can be reached by the individual only when he has overcome or abandoned the involvement of his mind in the world process and his attachment to the absolute separateness of his individual human consciousness.

The existentialist dictum that existence is prior to essence is best illustrated by the Indian doctrine of reincarnation or rebirth. The popular but erroneous description in the West of this doctrine as the "transmigration of souls" makes it difficult if not impossible for the European mind, accustomed as it is to the Christian belief in an unchangeable soul or to the Aristotelian assumption of the existence of rigid substances, to understand how the Hindus can believe that a man's soul can reincarnate in an animal. However, this popular belief of Indian religious followers has a profound philosophical nucleus: there exists no definite essence of "manhood" (or man's soul) in the individual nor a definite substance or essence in anything else. The life of an individual, or indeed of any other living being, is a dynamic and progressive process of self-realisation of a will to live, and to experience, which in its every single act of volition creates or modifies its character and nature in exact proportion to the gravity of the act. The sum total of manifest and latent volitional acts and tendencies may appear human, subhuman or superhuman, but it is never fixed forever: it is fluid and ever-changing, although the changes may for long periods be so small that they allow a temporary relative stability of character. But basically a man is what he has been choosing, which means that he is fully responsible for what he is and for what he experiences. In the latter case it is so because he is not faced with a world which is objectively what it appears to be to his consciousness, but his consciousness is selective, picking out perceptions of the world which correspond to his character or essence.

Three further preoccupations of modern existentialist philosophy—despair or dread, death and freedom—have also been of constant concern in Indian thought. Despair is voiced in all Indian systems, chiefly in terms of the suffering or unsatisfactoriness of life in its limited individual form. In the long run all volitional actions of the individual are condemned to personal frustration, although temporarily they may make sense: the Indian view allows some space for calculated volitional actions to bring about desirable results as it does not see the world as a hostile alien reality, but as the result of the sum total of volitional actions of all individuals who then are faced with those parts of it which they helped to form by their own acts. But with the prospect of, virtually, a never-ending and therefore, in the last instance, repetitive world process in which the individual participates in a sequence of successive lives, the individual existence finally loses all its meaning and sense. Frustration, disgust and despair are the result. And death is seen as yet another interfering and unavoidable occurrence which is frustrating in its senseless repetitiveness. There is no serious question, in Indian thought, of choosing death as an act of freedom and escape, for in the Indian view death means only a change of scene for the life of the individual, and the veiling of his memory. When this situation is recognised and understood by him, death is then a strong reminder to transcend his limited existential situation.

This now is where the question of freedom and its conception in Indian thinking presents itself with full weight. Generally speaking Indian philosophy is not preoccupied with freedom as a philosophical problem at all. It follows from a study of Indian systems that all of them (apart from an early deterministic school known only from references in early Upaniṣadic and Buddhist texts) assumed some kind of freedom of choice between various courses of action in concrete situations and a certain measure of freedom in choosing the course of one's life in general, such as a particular worldly career or the life of a recluse or wandering philosopher.

The volitional actions of an individual were closely dependent on the state of his knowledge, experience and intelligence, but even with respect to these personal qualities of an individual's character he was free to influence and finally determine the direction in which to go. In other words, the individual was always creating and forming his essence. If he did not exercise this freedom of his and did not cultivate the intelligence needed for it, he would, paradoxically, make a free choice of giving it up. As a result, the stream of life of the individual would continue on a sub-personal level, following its blind, inherent urge to live more on an instinctual basis, and a subhuman form of life might follow after the death of the individual.

The crucial and supreme act of freedom in the sense of a final choice may occur in the life of the individual only when his understanding of his existential situation has reached a high level and he takes the decision consciously to direct or try to direct, from now on, every further step in his life in order to master and finally transcend its limitations: in other words he becomes a practising Yogi. This is the Indian counterpart of the existentialist conception of the "authentic existence".

When brought to completion, a Yogi's achievement is supposed to be equivalent to absolute freedom from all limitations of a personal or individual form of life or, with some schools, to complete freedom from what we know as existence altogether.

At this point there appears the question of transcendence and its role in Indian philosophy as compared with existentialism. It does not matter, for our purpose, whether it is looked upon as "Transcendence" in the sense of a higher metaphysical reality or merely as some sort of experience which transcends the intellectual capacity of man to express and describe it conceptually. European existentialist philosophy simply stops at this point, which has different consequences for different existentialist philosophers as was described earlier in this chapter. In the Indian tradition, however, the experience or the achievement of transcendence is regarded as the final solution of the riddle of existence for the individual and much space is given to its interpretation and to attempts to describe it, even if only negatively.

The only way to the achievement of the experience of transcendence is individual Yoga practice of some kind and in the course of centuries several methods of Yoga practice have been elaborated in India by various schools. Some of them were so intent on the final achievement that they limited the philosophical or doctrinal part of their work to a bare minimum, and thorough and extensive elaboration of various aspects of the practical method of training and the way of life which should go with it formed the bulk of their teachings. This feature is best illustrated by early Buddhism. Also Patañjali's Yoga system is concerned predominantly with Yoga practice and progress and very little with philosophy.

It has been a special feature of Indian philosophy that the process of elaborating a specific Yoga path within, together with, or as the chief object of a philosophical teaching has always remained alive and has been demonstrated recently by the work of the widely known Indian philosopher and Yogi Aurobindo Ghosh.

The situation in the Western world is more complicated. Existentialism, phenomenology and various schools of psychoanalytical psychology are not yet generally accepted as indications of a new orientation of the Western mind. But many of their tenets and discoveries have become common property and a profound change in the Western attitude to the problems of existence and its meaning has undoubtedly been initiated. It is significant in this context that the above-mentioned schools have so many points in common with Indian attitudes, views and methods. At the same time direct interest in and preoccupation with Indian thought and Yoga are steadily growing.

Perhaps this development points to an inevitable and undoubtedly very desirable reconciliation of the traditions and cultures of the world. Its possibility has been greatly enhanced ever since the notion of the superiority of the European Christian tradition and Western materialistic civilisation started rapidly diminishing.

## CHAPTER II

# THE NATURE OF THE WORLD. A SURVEY OF INDIAN COSMOLOGY

Although man has always occupied a central position in Indian philosophy and although the primary concern of Indian thinkers has been the problem of his destiny as an individual, together with the question of the effect of his actions on his future and the possibility of a final breakthrough into the realm of absolute freedom, the world as the stage on which this drama of man's search is taking place has also received due attention.

The oldest source of information about Indian views of the world is the Ṛg Veda (literally, knowledge in verses), an extensive collection of religious hymns which used to be—and indeed still are—sung by Indian priests during religious ceremonies. These hymns comprise the reactions of the Indian mind to its encounters with experienced reality, both external and internal, that is, with the strange world of things that we perceive around us and with the mysterious world of mental processes that we sense inside ourselves. They were composed long ago, certainly before 1000 B. C., but many of them perhaps around 1500 B. C. and some of them even earlier. Some of the ideas expressed in these hymns certainly come from an even remoter past.

According to Indian tradition the Vedic hymns were transmitted to the people by ancient sages who were, "in their hearts", in direct contact with the Transcendental Reality, the Absolute, the direct source of all knowledge and of all existence (see the verse line "the sages, searching in their hearts with wisdom", RV 10. 129. 4). On the other hand Western scholars believed until recently that the Vedic hymns were produced by the creative imaginations of poets who through personification turned natural phenomena into a Pantheon of gods and paraphrased natural processes into a kind of popular physics and astronomy.[1] Despite their basic disagreement both these

1. The view that the Vedas are "imaginative creations of poets" was expressed by A.A. Macdonell, *Vedic Mythology*, p. 5 (1897). We find

views, the Indian traditional and the modern Western, imply that the knowledge put into the Vedas originated as the creation of a specially gifted élite who composed the hymns for the benefit of others in a language which the people of the time could understand and in a form which would make a deep and lasting impression on their minds. This is an important point. The use of the hymns during religious ceremonies secured their frequent repetition and therefore preservation in the memory of the officiating priests, and also their availability to the people who listened to them while taking part in the service, in a time when writing was unknown.

In the last two decades the modern Western view of the origin and meaning of the Vedas has changed considerably and has admitted a deeper explanation for them, thereby getting nearer to the Indian traditional view. It is now possible to express the view that the Vedic hymns convey their authors' recognition of a truth or reality which has a timeless and general validity and is, at least, a part of the world process. In other words, one can say that the Vedas contain real knowledge—as modern sciences do—only they express it in their own specific way. The mythological language of the ancient religious mind is different from the rational language of the modern scientific mind, but either of them is capable of expressing abstract knowledge, such as natural laws which are the results of precise observation (of recurring natural and astronomical phenomena) or profound concepts with philosophical significance, like that of infinity or that of morality, both of which are the results of observation as well as of intuition and precise thinking. Both languages use symbolism to convey the meaning, although their respective sets of symbols are of differing kinds.[1]

the same idea in one form or another in works of most scholars of previous generations like Oldenberg, Hillebrandt and Deussen. Even the Indian scholar S. Dasgupta seems to have echoed this view (especially Deussen's words about Vedic gods being "Produkte kindlicher Imagination", *Allg. Gesch. d. Phil.*, 1, 1, p. 79-4th ed. 1920) when he wrote: "The Vedic poets were the children of nature", *A Hist. of Ind. Phil.* I, p. 17 (1951).

1. The changed attitude of scholars has been appropriately voiced by Jan Gonda : *Die Religionen Indiens I, Veda und älterer Hinduismus*, Stuttgart 1960, pp. 23-24 : "Ein vedischer Mythus ist weder eine Dichtung

This implies that the authors of many or most of the Vedic hymns expressing these higher ideas were no mere primitive bards with the gift of imagination, but mentally highly advanced individuals with a developed capacity for observation and an intelligent grasp of realities, both external and internal (physical and psychological). If they were not just naturally gifted poets, they must have had some form of education or training behind them which had cultivated their minds to that level. Already during their time they were venerated as sages and their reputation as such has been preserved in India. We may regard them as the early representatives of a movement that incorporated a way of discipline and a method of cultivating the mind that later became known as Yoga (see chapter 5).

We shall now turn our attention to those elements of the Vedic myths that provide information about the world and its nature. A fragmentary, but most interesting picture emerges from their examination.

First there is the idea of Infinity which appears in the Ṛg Veda in the person of the goddess *Aditi*. She has several aspects, but one of them is that of free, limitless space. This means that the idea of the boundlessness of the universe current in later systems of Indian philosophy (especially in Mahāyāna Buddhism) had already found expression in the Ṛg Veda. But while the space through which we move is referred to in the later texts as ākāśa (meaning also ether), *Aditi* combines in herself also the aspect of "inner space" (*antarikṣan*, RV 1,89, 10). This is a dimension or dimensions in which gods and other spiritual beings dwell. It is at the same time the dimension of conscious-

noch eine populäre Physik, weder eine primitive Kontemplation noch eine embryonale Philosophie, obwohl sein eigentliches Wesen in der Regel mit Elementen von Dichtung und Welterklärung durchsetzt ist. Ein vedischer Mythus drückt in der Form einer in der zeitlosen Vergangenheit oder gerade im Zeitlosen sich abspielenden Erzählung von einer mit Macht geladenen, als real empfundenen, meist einmaligen Begebenheit (die sich in der Zeit, in der Natur oder im Ritus, oder auch im Ritus und dadurch in der Natur wiederholt) eine ewige Wahrheit aus, eine Realität, der die tatsächliche Wirklichkeit entspricht. Er beschreibt und deutet ein für den Menschen, der an ihn glaubt, wichtiges Weltgeschehen. Die stete Wiederholung des mythischen Ereignisses ist das, was sich in Welt und Kosmos immer wieder begibt."

ness and it also, of course, bears the characteristic of boundlessness or infiniteness. Thus *Aditi* comprises everything, being called the mother and father of all the gods and of all that which has arisen in the past and will ever arise (RV 1, 89). She is the all-embracing multidimensional and infinite element which is the basis of the manifested universe, sometimes called Mother Nature,[1] and she is also the transcendental light of consciousness.

So the infinity of the universe was understood in those days not only in its physical aspect, but also in the sense of the infinity of consciousness. The physical and the mental were felt to be present together in everything and to be inseparable. Or, in other words, the conceptual abstractions of mere spatial and corporeal extension on the one hand and of purely mental processes on the other had not been developed. Consciousness in one form or another was inseparable from any part of existence or from existence as a whole and simply represented its deeper dimension. Infinite space, therefore, was not entirely empty, but contained the latent (mental) seeds of all that was to come.[2]

Next, the manifested aspect of existence is symbolised in the Vedas by *Varuṇa*, the male god of the shaped universe and of cosmic order. He is the son of *Aditi*, which implies that the

1. See S. Radhakrishnan's comment on *Kaṭha Upaniṣad* 2, 1, 7 in his *The Principal Upaniṣads*, London 1953.

2. From what has been said it is apparent that the previous Western interpretation of Aditi as the personification of an abstract idea of boundlessness or freedom (H. Oldenberg, *Die Religion des Veda*, 3. Aufl. 1923, pp. 202-204) does not explain her character. Interpretations of her as the personification of some partial natural phenomenon, such as "the endless expanse beyond the earth, the clouds and the sky" (M. Müller, *Vedic Hymns*, SBE 32, p. 241), "the earth" (Pischel, *Vedische Studien* II, p. 86) or "the daylight" (Hillebrandt, *Vedische Mythologie* II, p. 95) are quite inadequate. Macdonell's attempt to see Aditi as the personification of the quality of Varuṇa and other deities described as "sons of freedom" (*aditeḥ putrāḥ*) completely misses the point (*Vedic Mythology*, p. 122). Gonda's description of Aditi as standing for the idea of "Breite, Weite, Unbeschränktheit" in nature (*Die Rel. Ind.*, I, p. 84) is a step in the right direction. The dimension of infinite consciousness present in the concept of Aditi was pointed out by Aurobindo Ghosh (*On the Vedas*, ed. 1956, chap. XIII).

world in its manifested form sprang from primeval undifferentiated, multidimensional infiniteness.

*Varuṇa's* name can be interpreted as "encompasser"[1] and this is an apt description for the god of the world of things or phenomena. For the things or phenomena of the manifested world are merely surfaced structures or forms which are internally empty. The surface of a thing surrounds—"encompasses" —a section of space and only appears to be a solid object in its own right and this is the case with the entire universe whose essence is no other than primeval pregnant emptiness, although it appears in manifold forms. The world is thus not composed of separate and independent things made of compact substance or substances, but of substanceless, empty shapes, created by the "encompassing" movement or power within the womb of the infinite. *Varuṇa* therefore symbolises the surface of things, the visible world, the manifested universe.

As well as representing this "encompassing" movement *Varuṇa* also stands for all the regularity that distinguishes "cosmos" from "chaos", activity and growth from slumber. Indeed, the transition from the state of latent existence to the state of manifested universe proceeds in a way which can best be described as organic growth from within, governed by an inherent tendency which in the manifested world is detectable as "law" or "order", both "natural" and "moral", a tendency which, when discovered in operation, makes one feel or say that the way things are going is right. This tendency or force is called in the Ṛg Veda *ṛta* and *Varuṇa* is its guardian. It guarantees a balanced, "rightful" or "lawful" course of events in nature (both external and internal), thereby enabling the existence of the world. *Ṛta* applies to the regular motion of celestial bodies as well as to seasonal changes in nature and the regular sequence of days and nights. All natural phenomena are governed by it. (The implications of the concept of *ṛta* for man and his life will be dealt with in the next chapter.)

The world therefore has a deeper source than can be seen on the physical level, and its appearance and functioning are ruled by an impersonal law of nature which alone makes its existence possible. The nature of this deeper source and the mystery of

1. Cp. Macdonell, p. 28.

the origin of the world occupied the minds of the Vedic seers profoundly. The famous "Creation hymn" (RV 10, 129) describes the vision of the primeval situation when "non-being" and "being" did not exist, that is when the manifested, shaped world of things, which either are or are not, had not yet emerged. But a complete voidness or nothing is not conceivable, "no-thing" being only a negation or a taking away of something. Therefore the seer called that which he visualised as the source beyond being and non-being, "That One". Its attributes are self-sufficiency and inherent dynamism[1] from which it follows that the situation does not remain unchanged. The One manifests itself[2] in the dimension of being by the force of *tapas* (literally "heat") which is best rendered as "creative flame" (verse 3). It is also called, in its lower aspect, desire (*kāma*), the primordial seed of the mind which caused the first movement towards manifestation and created the polarity of being and non-being, of things which seem to be something, but are demarcated by empty space (nothing), both without and within. All this, the hymn asserts, was discovered by sages who searched with wisdom in their hearts.

1. *ānid avātam svadhyayā tad ekam.*

2. *ajāyata.* Although the Creation hymn has been quoted in full in many publications, it may be convenient to reproduce it here as well. The translation by Macdonell is included in *A Source Book in Indian Philosophy*, ed. by S. Radhakrishnan and Ch. A. Moore, Princeton 1957, pp. 23-24.

(1) Non-being then existed not nor being:
There was no air, nor sky that is beyond it.
What was concealed ? Wherein ? In whose protection ?
And was there deep unfathomable water ?

(2) Death then existed not nor life immortal;
Of neither night nor day was any token.
By its inherent force the One breathed windless:
No other thing than that beyond existed.

(3) Darkness there was at first by darkness hidden;
Without distinctive marks, this all was water.
That which, becoming, by the void was covered,
That One by force of heat came into being.

(4) Desire entered the One in the beginning:
It was the earliest seed, of thought the product.
The sages searching in their hearts with wisdom,
Found out the bond of being in non-being.

Since this hymn is considered to be one of the latest in the Ṛg Veda (although still prior to 1,000 B.C.), its author may have summarised in it views handed down from much earlier times. He gives clear expression to his uncertainty as to the origin of the universe and in this we can see the early progress of rationalism creeping into the Vedas: he asserts that gods appeared only after the creation of the world and then he asks himself who may know whence all this has arisen. Answering, he concludes that no one knows, perhaps not even he who surveys the universe from the highest heaven.

The origin of the world remains something of a mystery for everyone and therefore it seems that it is best dealt with in a language of mythological imagery which will satisfy an unsophisticated mind and also be obviously meaningful to poets and others who are capable of vision—but it does present, then, many many difficulties to our studious intellects. In one of the Vedic hymns which describe the origin of the world the creation is described as a cosmic sacrifice of a giant man (*puruṣa*—RV 10, 90). This image implies that the process of creation is one of producing the visible world out of whatever preceded it. There is no notion of a creation from nothing, by a creator or by any other agency, in the Vedas; the word they use for creation is *sṛṣṭi* which should be correctly translated as an "emerging" or "emanation". The idea that the *puruṣa* (philologically this word corresponds to the English "person") is the material from which the world is made through sacrificial transformation again implies that the primordial state of existence possesses the element of consciousness, mentality or

(5) Their ray extended light across the darkness:
But was the One above or was It under?
Creative force was there, and fertile power:
Below was energy, above was impulse.

(6) Who knows for certain? Who shall here declare it?
Whence was it born, and whence came this creation?
The gods were born after this world's creation:
Then who can know from whence it has arisen?

(7) None knoweth whence creation has arisen;
And whether he has or has not produced it:
He who surveys it in the highest heaven,
He only knows, or haply he may know not.

intelligence and that it tends to present itself as an all-comprising and self-sufficient structure graspable by the intellect only with the help of the concept of a personality which is the only complete structure man knows from without as well as from within.

The hymn says that the visible world is only one fourth of the *puruṣa* and that the remaining three fourths are celestial dimensions. Similarly, the visible man is only a smaller part of the reality of a person. His greater and subtler part is within, in the dimension of mentality.

In seeking further to understand and express the mysterious force which is the basis of the world, the Indian seers and thinkers arrived at another designation which was to govern Indian philosophical and religious thinking for many centuries up till the present day. This was the concept of *Brahman*. As the language of philosophy in ancient times was—as was already pointed out in this chapter—that of symbols and images, *Brahman* was first introduced as being the sun and all that the sun can stand for: in the first place as the revealer of the things of this world by its illumination, but also as the spiritual light by which the world of knowledge is revealed. From ritual hymns of the Vedas and from subsequent ritualistic texts (*Brāhmaṇas*) it is known that *Brahman* was also the designation for the "sacrificial formula" which was believed to be so powerful as to bring about the desired results of the sacrifice. This means that it was felt to stand for the mysterious magic power by whose might things could appear which had not been manifested before. Finally *Brahman* came to be seen as the hidden source of the universe, as the sole reason for the whole creation which was its manifestation. It is praised as the world's innermost essence and as such it pervades everything, underlies everything and, at the same time, is transcendent to everything. It is totally independent of all things and exists only by and through itself (*svayambhū*), while everything else depends on it. The whole world has emanated from it, is sustained by it and will return to it again. But while the world exists and *Brahman* sustains it by being present in it as its essence, *Brahman* nevertheless exists simultaneously in its transcendence, undiminished and unperturbed by the manifestation of the world.[1]

The elaboration of the doctrine of *Brahman* took several centuries. In the period following the age of the Vedic hymns (from about 1000 B. C. onwards) the priests were highly attracted to speculating about *Brahman*. But their writings lacked the freshness and inspiration of the Vedic hymns and are full of heavy mythological parables and ritualistic symbolism which makes a very artificial impression. These writings are called *Brāhmaṇas* and their main objective, besides teaching the art of sacrifice, was to establish the cosmic significance of sacrifice as a ritual act and to explain the meaning of all other religious ceremonies. The doctrine of *Brahman* was tackled in the *Brāhmaṇas* in a very laborious and tiresome way. It became clearer and more understandable in the gnostic and philosophical texts of the *Upaniṣads* whose language was less mythological and started developing a conceptual character. The *Upaniṣads* form the closing part of the Vedas and the bulk of them was composed approximately between 700 and 300 B. C. Although the doctrine of *Brahman* was clearly and fully formulated for the first time in the *Upaniṣads*, it may be said that the whole process of elaboration that led to this formulation brought nothing substantially new, but it reformulated the old Vedic teaching on the "One" and made it more generally known.

From this time on religious and philosophical thinking in ancient India became more and more conceptual and led finally to the formulation of philosophical systems in which logic, dialectics and speculation play a prominent part, and in which inspired creativity and vision, which were the source of Vedic and, to a great degree, of Upaniṣadic literature, are no more evident. But the material for further religious and philosophical teaching did not change and the ideas of the Vedas and the Upaniṣads were elaborated and systematically developed. Because of the variety of trends in the Vedic and Upaniṣadic teachings, different systems of thought could be outlined which became, in the course of time and through further elaboration, more and more remote from each other until at length they became mutu-

1. Textual references for pursuing the development of the concept of *Brahman* in the Vedas and Brāhmaṇas are given fully by Deussen, *Allg. Gesch. d. Phil.* I, 1, p. 250 ff.

ally entirely contradictory teachings although none of them ever ceased claiming to be the true, or even the only true, interpretation of the sacred Vedic tradition. This is particularly so in the case of two of these systems, the *Sāṅkhya* and the *Advaita Vedānta*, the latter being a monistic teaching and the former a kind of pluralistic dualism.

Another tendency of the post-Vedic time was to popularise the ideas of the Vedas and the Upaniṣads in works addressed to wide circles of people, and that is why they were incorporated in popular epic literature as "philosophical episodes"—as in the case of the famous *Bhagavad Gītā*, which is a part of the Indian national epic *Mahābhārata*,—or told in the popular mythological literature of Hinduism, in the *Purāṇas* ("stories of old"). This tendency in Hinduism was undoubtedly encouraged by the activities of non-brāhmanic movements, such as Buddhism and Jainism and other and less known philosophical, ascetic and Yogic schools, which disregarded the religious authority of the Vedas and propagated their teachings directly among people in defiance of the traditional attitude of the guardians of Vedic lore inherited from the past, the priests (Brâhmans).

In order to give a representative survey of Indian post-Vedic views about the universe, the cosmological ideas of the Sāṅkhya, Advaita Vedānta, Buddhism and Hinduism will now be described briefly. All these schools of thought or teachings hold the view that the world process is beginningless as well as unending. An absolute beginning of the universe or of the process of "cosmic becoming" cannot be found and an end to it is inconceivable. This idea cannot be found expressed in the old Vedic texts, but it is not inconsistent with them, either. The problem of the beginning of the world seems to have remained, in the Vedic texts, a vague, indefinite idea, for even when the beginning of world creation is described by some Vedic hymn, it is clear that it was not felt to be an absolute beginning, while the end of the world was never really mentioned.

The idea of the endless duration of the world process must already have been current during the time of the oldest Upaniṣads, if not earlier, but it was first clearly stated and described in detail in the Buddhist texts of the *Pāli Canon* (e. g. SN 2, 15, 20) whose origin dates from the fifth century B. C., and it was later systematically elaborated in the post-canonical literature of Buddhism, especially also in the *Abhidharmakoṣa* of Vasubandhu in the fourth century A. D. It is, of course, dealt with also in the works of the Hindu philosophical systems and extensively described and worked out into a world history in the Hindu Purāṇic literature.

According to this view which is so generally accepted in India the world undergoes periodic destruction and renewal. The period of the manifestation of the cosmos, which is extremely long, is followed by an equally long period of latency or chaos. The oldest Hindu literary formulation of this teaching is possibly the one found in the *Śvetāśvatara Upaniṣad* (5, 3 and 6, 3-4) and in the *Maitrāyaṇīya Upaniṣad* (6, 17). Here the work of creating and destroying the world is attributed to God who alone remains awake even during the period of rest of the universe, and who keeps the whole gigantic world process of creation and destruction going.

The Buddhist accounts in the Pāli Canon (e. g. in DN 1, 1) are more extensive than those in the Upaniṣads. They date from approximately the same time as or perhaps from an earlier time than the Upaniṣadic views and describe the periodic manifestation and dissolution of the world as a natural process to which even God (named by them always *Brahma*) is subjected. As is evident from the Pāli texts, the driving force that keeps the world going is the craving and active entanglement of beings in the world process. Consequently they are not able to remain in the unmanifested dimension for more than the period of rest. At the beginning of the new period of manifestation, the being with the greatest mind potential wakes up in the higher, spiritual sphere of the new cosmos (called *antalikkha*, which corresponds to the Vedic *antarikṣan*, the "inner space") and becomes God or *Brahma Svayambhū* (Pāli: Brahmā sayampabho) of the whole world period. Other beings then wake up and gradually fill higher as well as lower spheres of the world and assume that they have been created by the first being, Brahma.

The Upaniṣadic view is not so very far from this Buddhist conception. There it is indicated (Śvet. Up. 6, 4) that it is the actions (karma) of beings that cause God to keep creation going, a view which reappears in later Hinduism. But the basic difference remained. For Buddhists the world was a product of blind craving, for Upaniṣadic thinkers it sprang from the transcendental Divine source.

*   *   *

The Upaniṣads are products of several thinkers or schools of thought and therefore it is not surprising that their views on fundamental questions are not always consistent. Dichotomies and even disparities in their ideas are not difficult to discover and one of them concerns the status and role of God or the the Divine source. It later polarised, within Hinduism, in the two different systems of philosophical thought, the *Sāṅkhya* and the *Advaita Vedānta.* In the Sāṅkhya system the course of the world is an autonomous process whose basis is *Prakṛti* or Nature which produces the whole of the manifested universe, including its psychic phenomena. The material and the mental phenomena are of the same nature, the latter being the finer and subtler and the former being the grosser products of the evolution of *Prakṛti* from its primordial state of undifferentiation (*pralaya*). As the evolution of *Prakṛti* goes on, every successive evolute is grosser than the previous one, until the whole world is produced.

The primordial state of *Prakṛti* cannot be described in phenomenological terms, but is explained as a state of relative balance between the three tendencies (*guṇas*) which constitute *Prakṛti*; these are the tendencies of lucidity (*sattva*), energy (*rajas*) and inertia (*tamas*). The state of balance between the tendencies of *Prakṛti*, which causes *Prakṛti* to remain unmanifest, is not static but internally dynamic and it cannot last. When the balance is lost, the process of world manifestation begins with the appearance of the Cosmic Intelligence (*Buddhi*), often called the Great One (*Mahat*), as the first product of *Prakṛti*. It represents the original, lucid (sāttvic) state of the universe as pure intelligence which latently comprises all subsequent evolutes as seeds or latent ideas (*buddhis*). In the course of further evolution the *Mahat* or the Cosmic *Buddhi* produces the principle of individuation (*Ahaṅkāra*), a state of manifestation of the universe which is characterised by the separative effort of the three tendencies of *Prakṛti* which thus creates sets of conditions for the individual manifestation of latent seeds and ideas of the *Mahat.* These sets of conditions are of a twofold kind, according to which of the two *guṇas*—namely lucidity (*sattva*) or inertia (*tamas*)—predominates in them, while the remaining *guṇa*—that of energy (*rajas*)—is present in both of them as the driving force (also known as *prāṇa* or lifeforce).

The sattvic set of conditions when brought to manifestation represents mental processes that exist in the world as forces or elements which are in themselves impersonal, but constitute, in innumerable individual structures (concrete beings) their mental faculties: the mind (*manas*); five cognitive capacities (*buddhi-indriyas*): vision, touch, smell, taste and hearing; and five capacities for action (*karma-indriyas*): speech, grasping, movement, emptying and generation.

The tamasic set of conditions (known as *bhūtādi*) is manifested as physical processes in the world that are also sometimes called substances or essences, but actually represent basic physical energies. They are called in the texts *tanmātras*; five in number, each one of them tends towards a corresponding sattvic cognitive capacity whose object it forms when it reaches its gross-material stage of manifestation. The first element manifested from the tamasic set of conditions is the element of extension which is called ether (*ākāśa tanmātra*) and stands for what we call space. Its final or grossest manifestation is sound (*śabda*). The next element to be manifested is that of vibration ("wind" or "air" —*vāyu tanmātra*) which finally produces atoms and, in the grossest form of its manifestation, touchable objects. The third manifestation of *bhūtādi* is the element of form (*rūpa tanmātra*) which produces visible (coloured) shapes. The fourth is the element of fluidity (*āpas tanmātra*), responsible for objects which can be tasted, and last comes the manifestation of the element of density (*kṣiti tanmātra*), which tends to produce objects that can be smelled. Structural combinations, in different proportions, of these essences or physical forces make up the individual things and objects of this world.

Although this process of world manifestation goes on without any impetus from a superior agent, such as God, it is not a mechanical process going on for its own sake, but rather it goes on for the sake of *Puruṣa* (Spirit) who is not a God Creator, but an enchanted onlooker. *Puruṣa* thus represents, in the Sāṅkhya system, the immaterial principle in the world, like *Brahman* in the Upaniṣads, but one that is entirely passive. He does not do anything and remains, in essence, eternally pure. Yet he becomes involved in the world process like a cinema-goer who forgets that he is not a party to the action going on on the screen and gets involved in and absorbed by it.

There are many *puruṣas* watching the performance (acting, as it were, as catalysts in a chemical reaction) and *Prakṛti* outlines the spectacle for them. Without them the world process would be unthinkable.[1]

* * *

The system of Advaita Vedānta claims to be the truest interpretation of the Upaniṣadic tradition and indeed it seems to be a more logical outcome and elaboration of the Upaniṣadic speculations on the emanation of the world from the *Brahman-Ātman* ( Tait. Up. 2, 1 ) or from the primordial unity ( Chand. Up. 6, 2, 2 ) than the Sāṅkhya system with its dualism.

The great philosopher Śaṅkara ( 788-820 A.D. ) undoubtedly believed that his advaitic (nondualistic) interpretation of the Vedic tradition was correct and consistent and so do many Hindus nowadays. Through the Ramakrishna Mission promoted in recent times by Vivekananda's activities and written work, the advaitic philosophy of Vedānta became known and influential in Western countries also, wherever Indian religious

1. Every book on the history of Indian philosophy has a treatise on Sāṅkhya; quite often the Sāṅkhya system and Patañjali's Yoga are treated together (e.g. by O.Strauss, H. Zimmer and S. Dasgupta) which cannot be looked upon as being quite correct. The following selection of monographs may be found useful to study :

R. Garbe : *Die Sāṃkhya-Philosophie*, 2. Aufl,, Leipzig 1917.
,, *Sāṃkhya und Yoga*, Strassburg 1896 .
A.B. Keith : *The Sāṃkhya System*, Calcutta—London 1918.
S. Dasgupta . *Yoga Philosophy*, Calcutta 1930.
E. H. Johnston. *Early Sāṃkhya*, London 1937.
A. Sen Gupta : *The Evolution of the Samkhya School of Thought*, Patna 1959.
G. J. Larsen : *Classical Sāṃkhya*, Delhi 1969.

and philosophical ideas and an interest in Yoga had taken hold.[1]

According to the philosophy of Śaṅkara, the Ultimate Reality is the *Brahman*, an impersonal, or more exactly, suprapersonal, principle of all existence which transcends all categories of description and understanding and is therefore described, as early as in the Upaniṣads, as non-existent (Tait. Up. 2, 7) and unknowable (Bṛh. Up. 3, 4, 2). However, it is also the cause of everything that exists and that is known as the world.

In the absolute sense only *Brahman* really exists, because it is beyond change, beyond time and beyond space, and has therefore no beginning and no end. The world exists in time and space and undergoes periodic creation and destruction and so from the standpoint of the Ultimate Reality its existence is entirely illusory. It is real enough only for the limited consciousness of individual beings living in the world. But illusory though it is, the world is nevertheless not non-existent (non-existence being, in one sense, a special attribute of *Brahman* and expressing its transcendental and ungraspable character), because its source and creator is Brahman itself whose reality guarantees the existence of the world.

But of course, the nature of the *Brahman* as creator or eternal originator of the universe is already a substantial step removed from the ultimateness of the *Brahman* in itself (*Nirguṇa Brahman* —*Brahman* without qualities or attributes). The notion of the *Brahman* with attributes (*Saguṇa Brahman*), such as that of a creator, is meaningful only from the limited point of view of an individual consciousness in this world. Conceived in this way the *Brahman* with attributes can be known as the personal God —as *Brahmā* the Creator or *Īśvara* (the Lord). And that is how he is described and addressed in many passages in the Vedic scriptures.

The capacity of creator of the universe does not endow *Īśvara*, as it does the Judaeo-Christian God, with the power to create a world once for all and then draft a plan of salvation

1. One of the contemporary popular expositions of advaitic cosmology was given by Paul Brunton, *The Hidden Teaching Beyond Yoga*, London 1941, and *The Wisdom of the Overself*, London (date not given).

and final transfiguration for it. For even in Śankara's system the periodic manifestation and reabsorption of the world into its source is a never-ending cyclic process. But because neither the *Brahman* as Lord the Creator (*Saguṇa Brahman*) nor the *Brahman* in itself (*Nirguṇa Brahman*) can be thought of as being under the compulsion of some natural law of necessity in bringing forth this periodic creation, Śankara, following Bādarāyaṇa, the first known teacher of the vedāntic tradition, explains this activity as being the result of a divine creative game (*līlā*).

As in the Upaniṣads, the creation of the world is described by Śankara as an emanation (*sṛṣṭi*) from *Brahman*. It proceeds in stages, representing a progressive process of "condensation" from subtle to gross constituents of the world. The first element to emanate from *Brahman* was space (*ākāśa*) thought of as ether, and then followed the four familiar elements constituting the so-called material world: the "wind" or "air" (*vāyu*), which may be called the element of vibration; "fire" (*tejas*), the element of heat and light; "water" (*āpas*), the element of fluidity or viscosity; and finally "earth" (*pṛthivī*), the element of solidity. The whole material world is made from combinations of these elements. But as the elements are emanations from *Brahman*, it must be assumed that every single thing as well as the whole universe is, by nature, *Brahman* itself in the state of temporary transformation, frozen, as it were, into the seeming solidity of matter.

At the same time, however, *Brahman* remains unchanged in its sublime transcendental unity, unperturbed by the periodic process of emanation and reabsorption of the world. Unlike Sāṅkhya, the Vedānta system regards the organic psychic phenomena as being of a different order from the physical universe, although, of course, having the same source, and they will be dealt with in the next chapter.[1]

* * *

1. There is abundant literature on Vedānta and again only a small selection can be given here :

M. Müller: *Three Lectures on Vedānta*, London 1894.

P. Deussen : *Das System des Vedānta*, 4. Aufl. Leipzig 1923, (English in Chicago 1912).

As has already been explained, the Buddhist view of the world and its nature does not differ substantially from the Brahmanic and Hindu conceptions, the chief point of divergence being that Buddhism consistently avoids the introduction of any conscious creator or transcendental (divine) creative source of the phenomenal world.[1] In fact, questions as to the origin of the world, as to whether it is eternal or not and whether it is infinite or finite were consistently answered by the Buddha with silence and his followers were advised not to waste time trying to solve them. The Brahmanic teaching about the creation of the world by the god *Brahmā* is entirely rejected and with an ironical undertone as if to indicate that it is a tale for simpletons.[2]

Despite this refusal of the Buddha to outline a cosmology, different passages of the Pāli Canon allow a picture of the

Kokileswar Sastri : *An Introduction to Advaita Philosophy*, Calcutta 1926.
Saroj Kumar : *Towards a Systematic Study of Vedānta*, Calcutta 1931.
H.v. Glasenapp : *Der Stufenweg zum Gottlichen*, Baden Baden 1948.
P. Hacker : *Die Schule Shankaras*, Wiesbaden 1951.
S. Radhakrishnan : *The Brahma Sūtra. The Philosophy of Life*, London 1960.
A. Hohenberger : *Rāmānuja. Ein Philosoph indischer Gottesmystik*, Bonn 1960.
S. M. Srinivasa Chari : *Advaita and Viśiṣṭādvaita*, London 1961.
M. K. Venkatarama Iyer : *Advaita Vedānta*, London 1964.
E. Deutsch : *Advaita Vedānta : A Philosophical Reconstruction*, Honolulu 1969.
E. Deutsch, J. A. B. van Buitenen : *A Source Book of Advaita Vedānta*, Honolulu 1971.

1. The problem arising from some later Mahāyāna views according to which *Śūnyatā*, conceived as "plenum-void" and identified with *Nirvāṇa*, is also the source of the manifested universe, is a more complex and specialised one and will not be discussed here, because there is no support for it in older Buddhist sources.

2. The views of early Buddhism concerning the nature of the world, the self and the problem of the final reality are best summarised in the *Brahmajāla Sutta*, DN 1, 1, where also the religious views of Brahmanic sects and teachers are criticised and their origin explained.

Buddhist view of the world to be made, and later Buddhist works are more explicit.[1]

According to the Buddhist view, the world is a continuous process of becoming brought about and constantly maintained by the mental volitional activities, conscious as well as unconscious, of all its inhabitants. Instead of a divine creator it is the desire to live and to experience which leads on the one hand to the perpetuation of individual forms of life, including man, and on the other to the periodic renewal of the world as the stage for life's processes to manifest themselves on.

The cause of the world is, therefore, mental: the will to live of individual beings. And in a way it could be said that the world is of mental character and does not exist at all apart from the individual. The Buddha is reported to have said: "I declare, friend, within this fathomlong body with its perception and thinking there lies the world, the origin of the world, the cessation of the world and the path leading to the cessation of the world."[2] But the old school of Buddhism (*Theravāda*) did not follow the possible metaphysical implications of this statement. Besides, it was not made by the Buddha as a metaphysical statement about the nature of the world, but as a hint to the effect that the final solution of man's quest for truth was not to be found in the outside world, but within himself. Although the world of an individual is necessarily subjective, it obviously overlaps with the worlds of other individuals and so the Buddhist texts of the Pāli Canon always refer to the world as if it were one structure inhabited by various beings. Moreover, individual beings are looked upon as structures composed of impersonal elements and lacking in any permanent mental basis, as will be shown in the next chapter, so that again the subjectivity of an individual's perceived world has no ontological bearing.

1. Even so, they do not add much to the oldest material which can be collected from the Pāli Canon, but chiefly develop and systematise it, as Vasubandhu in the *Abhidharmakośa*. An analysis of the Buddhist cosmology was given by W. M. McGovern, *A Manual of Buddhist Philosophy*, I, London 1923.

2. Api cāham āvuso imasmiṃ yeva byāmamatte kalebare saññimhi samanake lokañ ca paññāpemi lokasamudayañ ca lokanirodhañ ca lokanirodhagāminiṃ patipadan ti.—*AN*, PTS ed. 4, 45, 3—vol. II, p. 48.

In any event, the building stones of the world are described in thc Buddhist texts objectively and they are the familiar four elements known to us already from other systems: solidity or inertia ("earth"), fluidity or cohesion ("water"), heat or radiation ("fire") and vibration ("wind" or "air"). They are dynamic forces of nature and their combination produces the world of things and surroundings for beings to live in as well as their material bodies, whether they live on this earth or elsewhere in the material world or in "spiritual" (="fine-material") spheres of the universe, such as "hells" and "heavens".

The world appears to exist in space which tends to be viewed as infinite, although its character is again conceived in a way which does not quite allow real existence to be ascribed to it. From later sources it is clear that Buddhism has assumed the existence of innumerable world systems with innumerable living beings inhabiting them. And the whole world process with its periodic manifestation and destruction goes on ceaselessly; no beginning can be discovered, and an end to it is unthinkable. This does not necessarily mean that the world process is constantly going "ahead" to something new. Rather it seems that the texts conceive time to be cyclic and so the world process also is a cyclic movement, a constant regrouping of its elements (like in a kaleidoscope).

Each world system is divided into three spheres or existential planes, the highest being without forms (*arūba vacara*): only mental processes are going on there and it is often called the "immaterial sphere". The second one is the sphere of forms (*rūpa vacara*), often called the "fine-material sphere". Both these worlds, which have further subdivisions, are inhabited by spiritually highly-developed beings who possess deep meditative states of mind.

The third region is called the sphere of desire (*kāma vacara*) and it includes the visible universe and the lower and higher regions known in religious systems as hells and heavens. The sphere of desire has five or six divisions which in turn have further subdivisions. The best known representation of this sphere is the Tibetan "Wheel of Life" whose simplified scheme looks as follows:

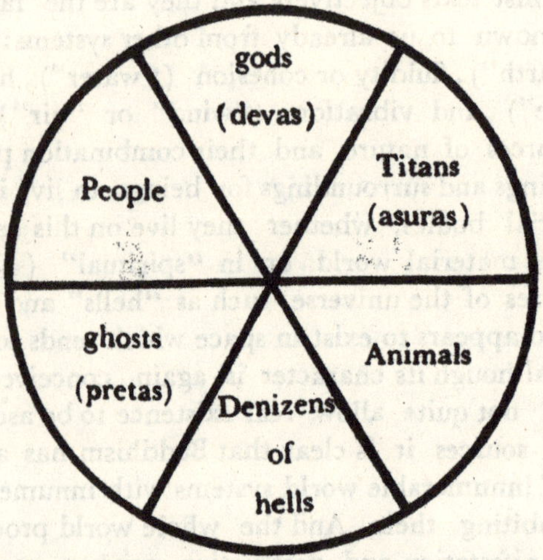


Some of these regions partly overlap and a limited communication between them is taking place, like that between *devas* and *asuras* and that between people and animals. Contacts between the inhabitants of other spheres are less frequent or even exceptional.

The sphere of gods (*devas*) is inhabited by all the deities of popular Hinduism and by the gods of the Vedic Pantheon, in different subdivisions. *Brahmā*, the highest God and "surveyor" of the universe, can manifest himself in any of the six spheres of *kāma vacara*, but his home region is the lowest subdivision of the sphere of forms (*rūpa vacara*). The fact that God is not granted the capacity of creator of the world—apparently a criticism of the current popular belief and of the prevalent Brahmanic teaching expressed later in various writings, especially in the Bhagavad Gītā and in the Purāṇas—is not really a Buddhist innovation, but is in line with the higher speculative tendencies of the Ṛg Veda (as expressed in the Creation hymn, RV 10, 129) and is also found in the post-Buddhist orthodox systems of Hindu thought such as Sāṅkhya, Patañjali's Yoga and Pūrva Mimāṁsā.

The *asuras* are usually called demons, but the word Titans may better express their character as conceived in Indian mythology, which has some points in common with the mythology of ancient Greece. Ghosts are described as beings who passed from the human world and have not yet found rebirth elsewhere, as their name (Saṁskṛt: *preta*, Pāli : *peta*) indicates. Their region corresponds to the Christian purgatory.

As has already been stated, there are innumerable world systems and they seem to have a kind of spherical spatial shape (one is even tempted to say: rather like Einstein's spherical universe). As a result, three neighbouring world systems create an intermediary dark region which does not belong anywhere and is inhabited by beings laden with the heaviest guilt.

The period of world duration being conceived of as unimaginably long, although not everlasting, the earliest sources of Buddhism already give an account of the subdivisions of world periods. One great world period (*mahākalpa*) is so long that the Buddha illustrates it with the following parable: if there were a solid block of rock, one mile long and equally broad and high, and once in a century a man passed by and his silk coat stroked the block, the whole block of rock would disappear, worn out by the strokes, before a great world period would come to an end.

Each great world period has four incalculable periods (*asaṅkhyeya kalpas*), the first one being the period of destruction (*saṁvarta kalpa*) in which the world regions of the universe, starting with the hells and ending with the world of *Brahmā* (the lowest subdivision of the sphere of forms), become gradually empty and then collapse in fire and general chaos. The beings from the destroyed world are reborn in other world systems, whose time scale is different, or in one of the higher subdivisions of the sphere of forms, if they are sufficiently mentally developed for them. The second incalculable period is one of rest for the world process (*saṁvarta sthāyi*) and the third one is a period of new evolution (*vivarta kalpa*) in which the world regions gradually appear again and are progressively inhabited. The fourth period is the time of relative world stability (*vivṛttāvasthā*) and of the historical development of mankind divided into twenty subperiods. Ten of them are subperiods of evolutional ascent and the other ten are subperiods of descent from the conditions of spirituality down to the material way of life. These subperiods alternate so that in the world history there is constant movement upwards to cultural and spiritual peaks and downwards to degenerate primitive conditions until at the end of the twentieth historical subperiod a new great world period begins.

* * *

The cosmology of Hinduism is neither uniform nor consistent. Views and myths from the Vedic hymns, Brāhmaṇas and Upaniṣads are, in modified forms and with new additions, scattered throughout the literature of Hinduism, especially in the epics (the Mahābhārata and partly also the Rāmāyaṇa) and in the Purāṇas. These works acquired their final form in the third or fourth century A.D. and influences of the Sāṅkhya system, of Yoga and of Buddhist ideas are obvious in them. The following is an attempt at a simplified picture of popular Hindu cosmology.

The world process has existed from beginningless time and will always continue. Its basis is the uncreated and eternal, primordial substance composed of five elements (earth, water, fire, air and ether) or else it periodically emanates from the transcendental Divine source or the Highest Divine being. The concrete images differ, but the most usual one is, that the Divine (which may be called *Brahman* or even *Siva* or *Viṣṇu*, as the sectarian followers use the name of their highest god even for the suprapersonal divine principle) first creates the "world egg" (i.e. the structure or basis of the world system) and then enters it or penetrates it with its divine power. Next the god *Brahmā* is brought to life to continue the work of creation and organisation of the universe in detail and to rule it. He creates the terrestrial world, heavens and hells with innumerable subdivisions and spheres of existence in which incalculable life forms appear.

One creation lasts as long as the life span of one Brahmā, who lives a hundred years, each year of his consisting of 360 days. One day of a Brahmā represents one small world period (*kalpa*), during which the world develops and goes through its history. At the end of a Brahmā's day the world comes to an end and during Brahmā's night there is a period of rest. One Brahmā's year represents one great world period (*mahākalpa*) which in turn consists of 1000 great ages (*mahāyugas*).[1] Each *mahāyuga* consists of four ages (*yugas*) in which mankind passes the peak as well as the nadir of its history. The happiest age is *Kṛta yuga* (which possibly means "accomplished age") with people enjoying long life, peaceful conditions and a high standard of spirituality. Next comes *Tretā yuga* and then *Dvāpara yuga* and in each of them the conditions worsen in all respects mentioned, although they are still far above present conditions in the world. (The names of these ages seem to have been derived from throws at dice, a cast of three and of two, respectively). Last comes the *Kali yuga* (the age of strife or dissension; sometimes "*kali*" is interpreted as "black, dark" and one speaks of the "dark age"). Conditions during the *Kali yuga* correspond to those which prevail in the world at present and they are expected to deteriorate even further. After a general collapse of civilisation a new *Kṛta yuga* will come.

The Purāṇas give exact calculations as to the duration of various ages, not only in a Brahmā's years, but also in the years of the gods, one year of theirs being 360 human years. Therefore it is possible to make the following timetable of the periods of one creation:

| | |
|---|---|
| Life span of one Brahmā: | 100 years of a Brahmā |
| | 864,000 million years of the gods |
| | 3,110,400 million human years |
| One day of a Brahmā: | 1 *kalpa* |
| | 1,000 *mahāyugas* |
| | 12 million years of the gods |
| | 4,320 million human years |

An equally long period is allowed for the night of a Brahmā, during which the universe is absorbed in him and he is asleep.

1. One kalpa is also divided into 14 *manvantaras* or "ages of Manu", each of them being presided over by one particular father of mankind or "Manu"; the present age is under the rule of the seventh Manu of this *kalpa*, who is called Vaivasvata. A.L. Basham thinks that the whole system of Hindu cosmology is an imperfect synthesis of more than one doctrine, particularly because *manvantaras* do not entirely fit into the system of *yugas*. See his *The Wonder that was India*, Fontana 1971, p.324.

| | |
|---|---|
| 1 *mahāyuga* (four *yugas*): | 12,000 years of the gods |
| | 4,320,000 human years |
| 1) *Kṛta yuga*: | 4,8000 years of the gods |
| | 1,780,000 human years |
| 2) *Tretā yuga*: | 3,600 years of the gods |
| | 1,296, 000 human years |
| 3) *Dvāpara yuga*: | 2,400 years of the gods |
| | 864,000 human years |
| 4) *Kali yuga*: | 1,200 years of the gods |
| | 432,000 human years |

According to the Purāṇic tradition the present Brahmā is in his fifty-first year of life so that the present creation recently passed the first half of its duration. The world is at present passing through *Kali yuga* which began in the year 3102 B.C. with the mythical destructive battle between the Āryan tribes on the *Kurukṣetra* which is described in the epic "*Mahābhārata*". As about one twentieth of each *yuga* at its beginning represents its "dawn", the present time is considered to be still relatively mild and peaceful; the really depressed period will start in about 18,000 years. When civilisation collapses entirely and *Kali yuga* comes to an end, a new *Kṛta yuga* will be initiated by a future saviour called *Kalki*.

When this whole creation reaches its end and the present Brahmā dies, the universe will be reabsorbed into the Unmanifest or the Divine source and an equally long period of a great cosmic night will follow. After that a new period of creation will start with the birth of a new Brahmā.

## CHAPTER III

# MAN, HIS ESSENCE AND DESTINY

If some modern existentialists feel that they have been thrown into a hostile and alien world or that the world they are condemned to live in is an unknown quantity, a mystery to them, in spite of all the scientific knowledge that man has accumulated about it, they seem to have overlooked that the other party in the world-man encounter, namely man himself, is an equally unknown quantity.

Man is indeed something of a mystery to himself, especially when he is an intellectually developed, thinking and inquiring person. It is at the thinking and inquiring stage of man's development that doubts and uncertainties prevail which only a few seem able to face throughout their lives or to resolve individually for themselves, perhaps by some act of direct, supra-intellectual cognition (such as a mystical vision or Yogic enlightenment). Most people avoid this unbearable uncertainty by accepting a faith, either in some traditional dogma like that of the existence of an immortal soul inside themselves or else in the modern "scientifically founded" materialistic theory according to which man with all the variety of his mental life is a product of chemical and electrical processes going on in his body, his individuality being an ephemeral and in itself unimportant by-product of the evolution of matter.

These are the two basic attitudes men have to the problem of their own status, whether they are fully aware of it or not. One or other of these attitudes is usually reflected in the works of philosophers and quite frequently of scientists as well, sometimes intentionally, but sometimes it seems that they have not arrived at a full realisation of the nature of the problem. The man in the street also adopts one of these attitudes, usually unwittingly. Sometimes both these attitudes strangely coexist in one and the same person.

Prior to the stage of intellectualism, and especially in the so-called primitive cultures, there does not seem to have been or to be any real doubts or difficulties as to what man and his destiny are. Everywhere in primitive and ancient cultures we find the conviction that although man is composed of elements and forces that are universal and belong to nature, he nevertheless is or possesses a personality that is an entity in its own right, and is in a way independent of the elements and forces of nature. This entity is—at least in the sphere of our European culture—mostly called "soul", and because in ancient cultures and primitive communities it appears to be of a complex nature, it was assumed by earlier explorers and researchers, who were used to the Christian idea of the soul as a unit, monad or compact indivisible substance, that the primitives and some ancient people believed in several souls coexisting in one body.

One rational explanation of this early and universally held idea of a soul which can survive the death of its physical body may readily be arrived at by conjecture: looking at a dead body, man may have reasoned that something must have left it, something that is closely associated with breath and is possibly of a shadowy character. During dreams, the soul leaves the body and wanders in this and other worlds, worlds where it is even possible to meet those who died in this world. The soul, although complex and immaterial, is obviously the real person, not the body. This is felt because the soul is the cause of bodily and other actions. And so the essential constituent of the soul is often felt to be the power of will—along with other powers, like that of warmth, that of being able to possess things, to give names and to communicate.[1]

Whether this and similar rational explanations are correct or not cannot be decided. They do help us to understand, from our intellectual point of view, the early stages of man's religious

1. Cf. J. T. Addison : *Life Beyond Death*, London 1933, p. 3 ff. The changing understanding and interpretation by scholars of primitive and archaic conceptions can best be seen when we compare synoptical expositions written several decades ago with present ones, for example :

E. Lehmann : "Die Religion der primitiven Völker" in "*Die orientalische Religionen*", Kultur der Gegenwart, Teil 1, Abt. III, 1, pp. 8-27 (1906),

V. Gronbech; "Primitive Religion" in "*Handbuch der Religions-geschichte*" 1, pp. 11-54 (1971, Danish original 1969).

conceptions, but it seems nowadays less plausible than ever that the "beginning" and evolution of religious ideas had some rationally explainable background. In particular the new attitude to the study of myths and symbols as reflected in the work of C. G. Jung and some of his followers has shown the need for a more open-minded and imaginative approach.[1]

In Vedic India the idea of man's surviving the death of his body seems to have been held as widely as in all other ancient civilisations, although the term "soul" is not here appropriate. A close study of the relevant Vedic hymns[2] shows that what was believed to survive was the whole personality of the departed one, including his bodily self (*tanū*). The personality was felt or conceived to be a complex structure whose directing constituent was the mind (*manas*). The mind was not only the "brain", but also the "heart" of the person; it comprised his thoughts, ideas, volitions and emotions, in short, his personal identity. Further constituents of the personality were animating vitality (*asu*); the vital cosmic force (*prāṇa*); the individual life process manifested in breathing (*ātman*); and various faculties constituting the experience of the bodily organism, such as hearing, seeing, blood circulation and solid parts of the body (like bones).

None of the constituents of the person actually belonged to the individual; all of them, including the mind, were regarded as cosmic forces (*devatās*) which had their respective abodes in the structure of the whole of the world (*idaṁ sarvaṁ*). Thus the mind belonged to the moon, breath to the wind, hearing to space, seeing to the sun, blood to water, flesh and bones to the earth. The names used for these cosmic forces do not convey to us their real character and have to be viewed as symbols. So the moon stands here for that sphere of the mind which in the individual remains mostly unconscious, but which possesses a high degree of lucidity in its cosmic dimension in which all experiences are preserved. Sometimes it is suggested in the Vedas

1. Cf. "Einleitung" by J. Rrytz Johansen ("Definitionen und Wissenschaften von den Religionen") in "*Handbuch der Religions geschichte*" 1, pp. 1-10.

2. E.g. RV 1, 140; 8, 89; 8, 100; 9, 113; 10, 14; 10, 15; 10, 16; 10, 57; 10, 58; 10. 90; 10, 154; AV 4, 34; 5, 30; 6, 18; 6, 120; 8, 1; 8, 2; 10, 15; 10, 16; 11, 1; 11, 2; 13, 1; 14, 2; 18, 2.

that the mind "goes to the waters" which has the same symbolic meaning of a cosmic reservoir of psychic images. (In this ancient symbolism can be discerned recognition of that essential constituent of the structure of reality as a whole which in Mahāyāna Buddhism is known as the "storehouse consciousness" (*ālaya vijñāna*) and which was newly recognised by C. G. Jung, who called it the "collective unconscious").

It would take us too far to consider the symbolism of the various other constituents of the person and their cosmic equivalents in the Vedas. Suffice it to say that the underlying idea of the essential identity of the forces constituting both the world and the individual can be clearly seen. The individuality of a person is centred in his mind (*manas*) which is the guiding, dynamic and selfconscious (as well as unconscious) force carrying his personal existence in its conscious part, whilst its unconscious part is linked to its cosmic reservoir. But there is also a constant interchange between all the other constituents of the person and their respective cosmic counterparts.

At death all constituents of the departed one merge in their cosmic counterparts and what remains of the individual is a mysterious shadow-like entity, a hollow double of him (a structure without contents), but this is immediately filled with its previous constituents which, purified and refined, emerge from their cosmic abodes and return into the personality structure. Thus the departed one is resurrected in the other world in a subtle form with all his constituents, including the bodily one. In other words, there takes place a transference or transfiguration of the person into a subtler and deeper dimension of existence.[1]

1. To present this picture it is necessary to supplement the scarce data of the Ṛg Veda and Atharva Veda with the information found in the Brāhmaṇas (e.g. *Ait. Br.* 1, 6, 13) and even in the earliest Upaniṣadic texts. However, a sufficient number of references is contained in the Ṛg Veda alone to justify this procedure. The hymns being a condensation of a much wider and more extensive set of ideas, views and experiences, their interpretation must go beyond mere listing of words occurring in them and their wide frame should be at least partly reconstructed.

Previous scholars tried in the main to confine their interpretations to what seemed to them to be explicit in the hymns, which resulted in

This conception should be noted for it shows that the transition from one world into another was not seen as the passing of an entirely identical person who merely moved to a different scene, but virtually as a new birth or a rebirth of that person in a different world or a different subdivision or dimension of the world. This was seen as happening repeatedly. Most or many of the deceased ones were believed to reappear first as what might be called "ghosts" (*pretas*, literally, the departed ones) in a world similar to this one, but not of equally gross material. Sometimes they could communicate with people in this world.[1] Some of them knew that they would die as *pretas* and appear in the world of fathers (*pitṛloka*) or go elsewhere. It appears that the multidimensionality of the world was clearly understood in the Vedic time and found not only a philosophical, but also a popular expression. A man

incomplete and fragmentary pictures. This was especially the case with A. A. Macdonell (cf. *Vedic Mythology*, p. 166 ff.). H. Oldenberg also split his descriptions, according to the three periods with which he dealt, into three separate works (*Die Religion des Veda*, *Die Weltanschauung der Brāhmaṇatexte* and *Die Lehre der Upanishaden und die Anfänge des Buddhismus*) without presenting an organic picture of the problem of the human personality and its destiny. A. B. Keith is not far from the same attitude in his *Religion and Philosophy of the Vedas and the Upanishads*, Harvard Un. Press 1925. All these scholars are also under the influence of evolutionism, and look on the ancient Indian religion as "primitive", and "evolving" with time the ideas that the 19th century's religious thinking in Europe held for the highly developed (such as the idea of a "soul" as a monad). In fact, the ancient religions in general, and the Vedic religion in particular, show an extremely high degree of knowledge of and insight into spiritual problems which, in the Vedas, are expressed in a poetical, symbolical and mythological language. Later centuries did, of course, develop conceptual and systematical language, but this does not imply that they reached a higher degree of understanding of religious matters. Conceptualisation of the issues quite often darkens the old insights rather than elucidates them for they were obviously drawn from the sources of inspiration which in systems developed later tends to get buried or even lost under a flood of words.

With respect to the Vedic conception of personality and its destiny, a somewhat more comprehensive and illuminating picture was given by H. v. Glasenapp in *Die Religionen Indiens*, Stuttgart 1943, pp. 80-85. J. Gonda hardly touches the problem in his *Die Religionen Indiens*.

1. Cf. the extensive passage on this theme in Oldenberg's *Die Religion des Veda*, pp. 555-566 (5th ed. 1970).

could reappear in a "dark, deep place", a kind of hell, or in the sphere of ghosts, in the world of fathers or in the world of gods. There are also some indications of the possibility of a departed man entering an animal life, or passing into a plant or joining the stars.[1] But a man could also enter other dimensions of existence while still in this living material body, which he could temporarily abandon. This normally happened when he was asleep or if he happened to faint (RV 10, 58). Dreams were memories from wanderings in other spheres. But it was also possible to develop the faculty of communication with higher spheres and beings in them, such as gods, during man's lifetime on earth (RV 10, 136).

The most widespread expectation man seems to have had in Vedic times with respect to his individual destiny after death was this : that he would join the fathers who had preceded him and would live a happy life with them, perhaps even in the company of gods, enjoying the fruits of his pious life on earth and of his posterity's ritual offerings. Only real evil-doers who had acted against what was right had to fear the dark place. The factor determining what was right was the same "law of balance"—*ṛta*—which guaranteed that water always flowed downhill, that day followed night, that there was regularity, reliability and harmony in the universe. *Ṛta* thus expressed everything that represented order (cosmos) as opposed to chaos in both the physical and the spiritual universe. This also implied the "rightful course of things" in man's actions—not only with respect to his fellow men, which is the domain of morality, but also in his relation to the whole of reality and to its higher aspects and forces, which is the province of religious practice, such as worship, offerings, all kinds of magic and ceremonial rites. (Both the English words "right" and "rite"—like the Latin "rectus"—correspond philologically to the Saṁskṛt word "*ṛta*".)[2]

1. See Keith, *Rel. and Phil. of the Vedas and the Up.*, pp. 415-6.

2. Although *ṛta* is referred to in numerous hymns in all its three aspects—the natural, the ritual and the moral—no single hymn is dedicated to it and its nature is never explained let alone analysed. It is therefore necessary to infer its universal character and effectiveness from a variety of hymns in which it is mentioned, e.g. RV 1, 1; 1, 144; 1, 156; 1, 189; 2, 9; 2, 23; 2, 30; 4, 3; 4 42 etc.

Offences against *ṛta* did not inevitably have unpleasant consequences in the life to come; most of them could still be remedied during this lifetime by appropriate action, such as the performance of a ritual or even a petition to those gods who were the guardians of the law, particularly *Varuṇa*. The most effective remedy, however, was to be constantly aware of *ṛta*, for this led to the avoidance of offences and their consequences (RV 4, 23, 8) and therefore, by implication, we can assume that it was believed that knowledge of the universal law gave man mastery over his own destiny or at least allowed him to influence its course. The full formulation of this belief appears only a few centuries later in the Upaniṣads together with an express formulation of the doctrine of rebirth.

The belief in repeated births in successive lives in this and other worlds and spheres of life may date from very early times even though it was not explicitly formulated then. The fact that the Ṛg Veda does not describe it clearly has often been taken as a proof that the belief did not exist at that time, but this is a wrong assumption. The Ṛg Veda being a collection of hymns and poems, no teaching or doctrine can be expected to be outlined in it fully or systematically. However, an awareness that man did not automatically become immortal when he entered the next world is clearly indicated in the hymns (e. g. RV 9, 113) and the continuation of the Vedic collections, the prose texts of the Brāhmaṇas, clearly express concern over the death man has to face again and again after his life on earth, if he does not attain immortality.[1]

1. *Tait. Br.* 3, 11, 86; *Kauṣ. Br.* 25, 1; *Śat. Br.* 2, 3, 39; 10, 1, 4, 14; 10, 2, 6, 19; 12, 9, 3, 12; 10, 4, 3, 10; The views of scholars differ on this point. Typical are the following ones.

Oldenberg was (favourably) inclined to admit the antiquity of the rebirth doctrine (*Die Lehre d. Up.*, pp. 24-26) for he recognised that the nature of the Ṛg Veda did not allow the use of *argumentum ex silentio* to disprove the existence of a doctrine of which at least some hints can be found.

Keith opposed it strongly, though not convincingly (*Rel and Phil.*, p. 570 ff.).

Deussen accepted the fact that the repeated deaths mentioned in the Ṛg Veda implied repeated births in the other world, but he stressed that this did not yet mean reincarnation in this world which was taught later

When the doctrine of rebirth emerges clearly in the Upaniṣads, it fully accords with the explanation of how the law of balance (*ṛta*) operates in human life and the law thus appears to be the basic force upholding moral order in the universe. No ruling divine authority is needed to back it. Man's destiny is formed by the quality of his previous deeds; good deeds bring good results, bad deeds bring suffering to the doer. The force of his previous actions also determines his character in future lives. "One becomes pure by pure actions, low by low ones."[1]

Although in the formulations of the doctrine of rebirth the role of action (*karma*) always receives the most emphasis, there are two further, and even more important, factors which shape man's future destiny and status. They are his knowledge and his previous experience. When man's physical organism dies and the life force departs from it, "he becomes a purely mental being; what is of mental nature, follows him; knowledge, actions and previous experience envelop him."[2] Here action (*karma*) is classified as being of mental character (*savijñāna*), like knowledge and experience, and we can conclude that already at this time of the older Upaniṣads the expression "*karma*" had two meanings (as it has in Buddhism and later Hinduism), namely "action" on the one hand, and "volition" meaning the mental

in the Upaniṣads (*Allg. Gesch. d. Phil.* I, 2, pp. 294 ff.—4th ed. 1920). This, however, is not the point. The heart of the question is whether the ancient Indian idea of afterlife envisaged its continuous duration in eternity after one earthly life or whether it envisaged man repeatedly dying and, consequently, being reborn, immortality being won only in special circumstances by special individuals. And the latter is undeniably the view of the Ṛg Veda. Being born again on this earth is not ruled out by the lack of direct reference to this view in the hymns and since it was clearly taught in the Upaniṣads, it must have been a current view in some circles long before. But for the philosophical significance of the idea of rebirth or the doctrine of transmigration the places of rebirth are not as important as some scholars thought they were, particularly as far as the rebirth on this earth is concerned. In all later expositions of the doctrine both Buddhist and Hindu, rebirth on earth is only one among many other possibilities.

1. *puṇyo vai punyena karmaṇā bhavati, pāpaḥ pāpena iti. Bṛh. Up*, 3, 2, 13.
2. *savijñāno bhavati, savijñānam eva anvavakrāmati; tam vidyākarmaṇī samanvārabhete pūrva prajñā ca. Bṛh. Up*- 4, 4. 2.

condition or determinant of action, on the other. The outcome of the volitional processes of the human mind, however, depends on the individual's knowledge and past experience and that is why these two factors are even more important than *karma.* Man's future is therefore shaped, according to this Upaniṣadic teaching, by what he has consciously and actively appropriated to himself in terms of knowledge (*vidyā*), by the general trend of his volitional tendencies (*karma*) and by what he has absorbed in the course of his life as his experience which then remains available to him as inborn intelligence (*pūrvaprajñā*) in future encounters with reality. Having then abandoned his old body, he creates for himself out of these mental constituents of his personality a new body which, according to the degree to which he has done away with ignorance, may be of a more beautiful shape than his previous one. It may be "like that of the fathers or the celestial beings or even that of the Lord of creatures (Prajāpati), of a Brahmā or of other beings" (Bṛh. Up. 4, 4, 4). It appears, however, that one lives in these other worlds only as long as the fruits of actions performed in this world last. When they are exhausted, one again returns to this world to start new work. (Bṛh. Up. 4, 4, 6).[1]

Various other parts of this and other Upaniṣads elaborate also on the occurrence of rebirth in lower worlds than the human one and on rebirth in this world as an inferior creature, such as an animal, or even as an insect in the case of previously wicked people.

The Upaniṣads are also more explicit about the nature of man's personality than were the Vedic hymns. It is, however, necessary to mention again the problem of the language of the texts as a medium for communicating the experiences, insights and ideas of their authors, and also to consider the whole nature of the Upaniṣads. They are not systematic treatises, but a collection of essays, dialogues and religious expositions of variegated origin, sometimes highly metaphysical, sometimes again mythological. Their language is not developed into a tool for precise conceptual inquiry into the nature of the experience of reality. The experience of reality is given in descriptive

1. Cf. Keith, *op. cit.* pp. 514-61.

terms chosen intuitively rather than from linguistic consideration of their possible exact meaning. Although this makes it difficult to interpret them conceptually, it does not diminish the profundity of their insights; for they are still capable of bringing about a deeper understanding beyond the reach of concepts just as it is possible to grasp the underlying meaning of an inspired poem even though it may escape full conceptual interpretation.[1]

The Upaniṣadic conception of man does not differ, basically, from what we know from Vedic hymns, but it adds a few more details to the picture and, most importantly, it attempts to grasp the innermost essence of his personality. He is still viewed as consisting of universal elements that leave him on death and return to their cosmic counterparts, but the part that remains of him is described in more explicit terms than in the Ṛg Veda. As we have already seen, what remains is his mental structure: knowledge (*vidyā*), volitional aiming or tending (*karma*) and previous experience or inborn intelligence (*pūrva-prajñā*). This mental structure which, although changeable, survives the body, is often called mind (*manas*; Bṛh. Up. 4,4,6), as it already was in the Ṛg Veda, or—newly—consciousness or "mentality" (*vijñāna*, Bṛh. Up. 4, 4, 2) which thus appears to be the name given to the whole mental part of man. What the Upaniṣad is getting at here is obviously what we would call "person", "personality" or "the structure of personality" with all its mental capacities but without its material counterpart, the body.

In another section of the same Upaniṣad the question as to what is left when a person dies is answered thus: "Name (*nāma*). The name is verily infinite." (Bṛh. Up. 3, 2, 13). The Saṁskṛt word "*nāma*", linguistically identical with the English "name" denotes all that is felt as constituting a personality, hence it could be translated as "character".[2] "Name"

1. A typical example of a scholarly interpretation insisting on purely historical-philological analysis is Keith's approach. Cf. particularly his piece on "The Supreme and the Individual Souls" in "*The Rel. and Phil. of the Vedas and the Up.*", pp. 551ff.

2. In later periods of Indian thought "*nāma*" is also used in the sense of 'substance" as opposed to "quality" (*guṇa*).

in ancient and archaic thought meant much more than it does today. It bore a magic relation to its bearer's personality and that is why here it may stand for it. (This meaning of "*nāma*" is retained also in early Buddhist thought.)

But this is only one part of the problem. When man dies, it is he who is "enveloped" in knowledge, volition and previous experience. His character or personality is thus only his shell. But who is he? The answer is *Ātman* (self): "This self, having cast off this body, removed ignorance, makes for itself another, newer and more beautiful form . . .".[1] *Ātman* is thus proclaimed to be the innermost essence, the real self of man.

We met *ātman* in the Ṛg Veda as one of the constituents of personality where it stood for the life force in the individual, manifested as breathing. But in the Ṛg Veda it very often designates the person himself and is also used as a reflexive pronoun which already indicates the meaning "self". In this connection it comes very close to meaning the "essence" of a person, called usually "soul" in Western religious terminology. In the Vedas *ātman* may mean the essence of a person, an animal or even a thing.[2] But since all the other constituents of a person—or of anything else, for that matter—were felt to be universal forces (*devatās*), so *ātman* had already in the Ṛg Veda the implicit character of universality, whether viewed under the aspect of a person's "breath of life" or as his innermost essence.

It is not surprising, therefore, that when *ātman* emerged in the Upaniṣads as man's true self, it was at the same time seen to be the self of everything else and of the world as a whole as well. From here it is only a small step to the identification of the *Brahman*, the transcendental cosmic source of the universe, with this *ātman*, or rather *Ātman*, the inner essence of man and all that exists. Thus two lines of inquiry, one proceeding by analysis of cosmic phenomena, trying to find their basis and source, and the other turning its attention to man in order to find out what he actually is in himself, meet here and find themselves facing the same mysterious and transcendental source of all being.

1. *ayam ātmā idam śarīram nihatya, avidyām gamayitvā, anyam navataram kalyāṇataram rūpam kuruṭe*... *Bṛh. Up*. 4, 4, 4.
2. For quotations see Deussen, *op. cit.* pp. 324 ff.

For the sages of the Upaniṣads, *Ātman* as the inner essence in everything is not a mere concept within the thinking mind. It is deeply felt that *Ātman* is the inner intelligence, the inner controller (*antaryāmī*) in all things, the unseen seer, the unheard hearer, the unthought thinker (Bṛh. Up. 3, 7, 1-23). When *Ātman* is experienced in this way, *Brahman* is reached as well and this means immortality. *Ātman* is the support of all worlds and all beings. It dwells in man's heart (in the innermost centre of his personality) and it is there that it can be directly experienced as *Brahman*. The human "heart" or centre of deep inner experience is thus a point of contiguity or of intersection where the Cosmic and the Individual meet, where *Brahman* and *Ātman* are one (Bṛh. Up. 3, 5, 1).

As long as man in his ignorance does not realize this, he can be only faintly aware of his true nature and is instead conscious rather of his individual self (*jīvātman*). But on reflection he can see that even in this limited situation he experiences different stages of consciousness which indicate and foreshadow the possibility of the unification of his superficial consciousness with his innermost essence, the universal *Ātman* or *Brahman*. In his everyday experience during his waking hours he sees himself living in a world that is external to him and he does not see the essential oneness. When he is asleep and dreams, however, he has a small private experience of a space and world around himself which is actually produced by his own mind just as the real universe is derived from *Brahman* or from the universal *Ātman*. When in a state of deep sleep without dreams, he acquires an even higher temporal experience, namely that of unification with the essence in which there is no duality and therefore no sorrow, only bliss. But he cannot take this experience back with him into his waking state. Only an aftertaste of bliss remains in him after a deep sleep (Bṛh. Up. 4, 3, 1-34). The full and uninterrupted knowledge of the Self (*Ātman-Brahman*) is known to the Upaniṣads as "*turīya*", the fourth state, and will be dealt with in the next chapter.

* * *

The post-Upaniṣadic development of Indian religious and philosophical thought is almost entirely dominated by the teaching of rebirth which gives Indian doctrines their specific character.[1] The next stage in the formulation of the teaching of rebirth was reached by Buddhism, which elaborated especially its ethical aspects. The law of *karma* represents, for Buddhism, a predominantly moral force in the universe. Strictly speaking, Buddhism has never denied the working of the universal law (known in the Vedas as *ṛta*) in the sphere of ritual and sacrificial lore and, of course, also accepted its validity as the law of nature. But in human life both these aspects of the universal law are subordinate to its moral aspect. This is brought about by the capacity of man to act consciously and use his knowledge of the law. It is then the motivation behind man's volitional activities and decision-making in combination with the degree of his ignorance or knowledge of how the universal law works that determines the final fruit of his actions. In its essence the law of *karma* in Buddhism is as impersonal and neutral a law of balance governing the world process as is the Vedic law of *ṛta*, but its effects within the process of human life appear to be of a purely ethical character.

According to the moral standard of man's desires, intentions, decisions, and actions, his character develops subsequently into a higher or a lower one. The level of his knowledge or ignorance and the quality of his consciousness are further factors which influence his actions and shape his character. He can then reach higher or lower stations on the scale of beings, becoming perhaps a god or even a *Brahmā*, or acquiring a subhuman status. If he preserves his human personality in his future life, his personality may still change widely in quality and level of intelligence. The environment into which he is reborn, as well as the events, opportunities and limitations in the course of his life so long as they are not the direct results of his actions during the present life, are also the consequences of his previous deeds and endeavours in past lives which have needed more time to ripen.

1. An exception to this is the teaching of materialists (*Cārvākas* or *lokāyatas*) who believed hat man was a product of four material elements like everything else. Life and the quality of consciousness were produced by the elements in the same way as "the power of intoxication is generated in molasses" (*Sarvadarśanasaṁgraha—Cārvākadarśana*).

According to this teaching every being is reborn after death in some subdivision of one of the six spheres of life (described in the previous chapter) in an appropriate form and with the pattern of his life determined by the character of his actions in previous lives. The human life is seen as the most important one, because in subhuman forms of life the sufferings or the struggle for survival makes it practically impossible for the individual being to influence his future destiny, while in higher or superhuman spheres he enjoys the results of previous good deeds and is little interested in anything else, as there is no pressing need for such interest. Only when the results of past bad and good deeds are for the most part exhausted both in subhuman and superhuman spheres, does the residual human *karma* bring the individual to a human birth once again and here he starts anew building up his bad or good—or, most frequently, mixed—*karma* for the future.

The sequence of lives in different spheres is not generally determined and, depending on the action of the individual, he may keep returning to a human rebirth for innumerable lives, or the spheres in which he is reborn may change frequently. The general pattern, however, seems to be one of slow ups and downs, as long as there is no conscious effort to influence one's career after an insight into the operation of the law is gained, Thus after a life full of bliss in super-human heavens he is reborn in the human world. As his character was shaped by previous experience of easily available pleasure he tends to take the pleasures of life for granted and as they are not readily forthcoming as they used to be, he starts pursuing them, and this gradually leads to the increase of selfishness and to ruthlessness, and the character finally acquires "beastly" or "devilish" features so that in the long run subhuman existences are unavoidable. During long periods of time filled with suffering in subhuman spheres of life, bad inclinations become gradually eliminated and when a human birth is again reached, the upward trend of the individual's character, resulting in an unselfish and decent life, will bring him eventually to higher worlds again and the whole story starts anew and may go on without end.

The beginning of this cycle of life is not conceivable: "A world without end is this round of birth and death. No beginning can be seen of those beings hindered by ignorance, bound by craving, running through the round of birth and death."[1]

Although without conceivable beginning, the round of rebirths (*saṁsāra*) can, however, be ended by an individual who acquires insight into the nature of existence and the law which governs it, abandons, as a result, the desire to live as he has done so far, and who then through his own exertion reaches final liberation, which is the only aim for which the Buddha is said to have preached his doctrine (see the next chapter).

But who, again, is the individual according to Buddhism and what is his nature?

In conformity with its pragmatic attitude, traditional Buddhism is silent on the problem of what is the essence of man, as speculations about the metaphysical nature of man do not help the aim of salvation. One should wait and see afterwards. What is given in the Pāli Canon is purely an analysis of the empirical constituents of the human personality as accessible to his present experience. The analysis describes man as composed of five groups or "bundles" (*khandhas*) of constituents as follows:

1. The "bundle" of corporeality (*rūpa khandha*). Corporeality is not an exact translation of the word "*rūpa*" which means "shape" or "form" and does not necessarily imply existence of "matter" in the philosophical sense. It is said to be composed of the same four elements or forces of nature as the world (see the previous chapter). Man experiences this part of himself as bodily awareness. On physical death it appears that man leaves his body behind so that his further existence will be without one, but in his experience nothing much is changed. He finds himself in another form, has another bodily awareness; only the change of his environment was more abrupt and far-reaching than the changes he had experienced during his previous life and so was the change of his bodily

1. See "*Some Sayings of the Buddha*" trans. by F. L. Woodward, London, repr. 1960, p. 181. The sources of traditional Buddhism do not present a systematic exposition of the doctrine, but quite extensive utterances about it are scattered throughout the Pāli Canon.

form or bodily awareness in comparison with the much slower changes that take place during our life when the body is growing old.

2. The "bundle" of feelings (*vedanā khandha*). Feelings are experiences of pleasure and unpleasantness or of neither or of indifference. They constantly accompany the individual's conscious life as its colour and undertone, but sometimes they are overwhelming and fill his entire experience for a brief moment. Being produced mostly by his reactions to his perceptions and thoughts, their pattern is almost constantly changing.

3. The "bundle" of perceptions (*saññā khandha*). The process of perceiving is experienced as sixfold, namely as perceptions of forms, sounds, odours, tastes, tactile or bodily impressions, and mental objects, such as thoughts, ideas, memories and images.

4. The "bundle" of mental processes or "formations" (*saṅkhāra khandha*). This group represents mental processes of a volitional character. It includes a number of both consciously and unconsciously active mental factors, such as instincts, urges, inclinations, desires, wishes, decisions and also such factors as attentiveness on the one hand and mental sluggishness or torpor on the other. It can be summarised as the sum total of mental qualities and faculties of a dynamic nature, usually called man's character, which also includes the conscious capacity for decision-making. The individual elements of this structural unit are of varied duration, from a passing whim lasting for a moment to a deep-rooted habit stuck to for years or to an instinct or a talent persisting through many lives. The whole structure is therefore constantly undergoing some change, while continuity is preserved not only during one life but throughout the entire sequence of lives of one individual.

5. The "bundle" of consciousness (*viññāna khandha*). Consciousness is the most important part of the structure of personality, penetrating all its parts in acts of awareness. There is no definition of consciousness in the Pāli Canon which would allow it any form of independent existence as a substance or a pure process. Rather it is described as a continuous process of being aware of forms, sounds, odours, tastes, tactile impressions and various mental objects or factors. It is never found without

one or more elements of the other groups constituting human personality (Sam. N. 22, 53) which are penetrated by it. Obviously, it covers "actually conscious" as well as "unconscious" mental factors which can exist as parts of man's experience only through the element of consciousness. In this sense consciousness (*viññāṇa*) is said to survive physical death, carrying with it the whole mental framework of the personality (*nāma*) which includes the other three mental "bundles" of constituents (*vedanā, saññā, saṅkhāra*) except the remaining one, the body (*rūpa*). However, a new body or form is again acquired immediately after death according to karmic dispositions and the surroundings in which the person appears. And so the structure of the personality "rolls on".

As there is a constant change within the structure, and the personality itself is viewed by traditional Pāli Buddhism as a purely phenomenal structural process (sufficiently described by the five *khandhas*) which does not possess any underlying substantial kernel (such as a soul or *Ātman*), there is no strict identity between successively reborn personalities, although there is a direct and uninterrupted continuity of the personality process. The reborn person cannot be described as being the same as the previous one, but he is not different from him, either (*na ca so, na ca añño*). And this description is extended to the description of personality within one single life in which a person can change beyond recognition both physically and in character, although the continuity is clearly preserved.

This conception of the personality, although complete from the empirical point of view, still leaves a certain residual feeling that there is something missing in the picture. This is so especially when the Buddhist way to liberation is described for it is done in terms of transcending the empirical personality structure as it is defined by the five *khandhas* and this results in an impression that the liberated person ceases to exist as soon as he dies. This view was already voiced several times during the lifetime of the Buddha who each time emphatically denied that he taught the final annihilation of the liberated one. Nor, however, did he teach a permanently existing and unchanging substratum, substance or essence existing within the personality. The nature of the liberated one, he stressed, was deep, unfathomable, to be understood only by the wise, meaning by a liberated one alone.

Yet about two or three hundred years after the Buddha's death this tendency to formulate conceptually what was the true nature of the personality resulted in a personalistic teaching (*pudgalavāda*). According to this school the person (*pudgala*) fully exists not only as a phenomenal structure, but also in the ultimate sense. They were anxious not to contradict the Buddha's own statements as preserved in the Canon and they did not identify the person with the experiencing self, which would mean accepting the existence of an individual soul (*jivātman*), or with an ultimate Self (*Paramātman*), which would bring them into agreement with Brahmanic conceptions based on Upaniṣadic philosophy. They only asserted the full reality of the "structural unity" of the person which is not in the five *khandhas*, is not outside them and is not identical with them either. They admitted that the person is undefinable and is fully known only by the Buddhas.[1]

* * *

Of the other schools of Indian religious and philosophical thought it is again Sāṅkhya and the Advaita Vedānta of Śankara which present us with two developed, but almost entirely opposite, conceptions of the human personality. As far as the question of the post-mortem destiny of man is concerned, all Hindu as well as Buddhist schools, systems of philosophy and individual philosophers until the present day accept the doctrine of rebirth or reincarnation based on the operation of the impersonal law of balance (now usually called *Dharma*, though virtually identical with the Vedic *ṛta*) which manifests itself in human life as the law of karma or the impersonal ethical order governing human affairs. Differences in the details are not of any consequence for the principles of the doctrine as they were first formulated in the Upaniṣads and elaborated in early Buddhism. Therefore we shall deal only with the teachings on personality in these two systems.

1. For further discussion of the *pudgalavāda* see E. Conze, *Buddhist Thought in India*, London. 1962, pp. 122-32; cf. also Keith, *op. cit.* 175-6.

Sāṅkhya can be classified as a philosophy of personalism within a broader framework of a metaphysical dualism. As we have seen in the previous chapter, the empirical personality of man in all its constituents including the mental ones is a product of the sattvic forces of *Prakṛti* and does not constitute a real person. It is thus only an elaborate and sophisticated puppet playing its part for the sake of the onlooker, *Puruṣa*, who is the real person and who by getting absorbed in the performance which he watches lends it the light of his consciousness, without which there would be no show.

*Puruṣa* is a pure spirit whose nature is consciousnesss (*cit*) This consciousness as an accompanying factor of every process that is going on in *Prakṛti* makes it into an experience, gives it a meaning and enables it to be taking place at all. Consciousness is therefore *Puruṣa* himself (or perhaps itself would be the proper word, for *Puruṣa* has no discriminative marks such as gender) and is not an impersonal element or process flashing within the individual structure of personality as is often explained in Buddhist commentatory literature. *Puruṣa* enables the empirical personality to become conscious and take part in the world process, but despite the fact that he identifies himself with the empirical personality like a spectator with the hero of the action on the screen during a film performance, he never himself becomes limited or tainted by the experiences of the empirical person. He is eternally free and pure, even though he has forgotten this fact.

Being of the nature of pure consciousness, which is never really experienced by the individual, empirical person, *Puruṣa* cannot be defined, perceived or known in any way. He is transcendent, although real and concrete. There is an individual *Puruṣa* behind every phenomenal person so that there is an indefinite number of *Puruṣas* in the universe. Sāṅkhya resolutely denies the possibility of one universal *Puruṣa* behind individual phenomenal persons, because their separate experiences such as births and deaths could not take place for them separately and at different times, but only simultaneously which, obviously, is not the case (*Sāṅkhya Kārikā* 18).

As was shown in the previous chapter, the empirical personality is composed of impersonal elements or forces which under the influence of the principle of individuation (*Ahaṅkāra*) mutually intersect, as it were, at many different points and these points of intersection are grouped into innumerable numbers of separate structures or concrete beings—of course not in their own right, but through the illuminating power of the individual *Puruṣas* behind them. When a structure is abandoned by a *Puruṣa*, its mental constituents disappear and it becomes a dead body which decomposes.

The process of "illumination" of the empirical personality by the *Puruṣa* is enabled by the fact that the mental constituents of the empirical personality are the products of the force of lucidity of Nature (the sattvic *guṇa* of *Prakṛti*). The sattvic *guṇa* has a certain affinity and receptivity towards the *Puruṣa* and as a result of being illumined by him produces *buddhi* or intelligence (both on the cosmic and individual level). Individual *buddhis* so resemble *Puruṣas* that the latter fail to see that they are different from them and accept everything that is happening within their *buddhis* and, consequently, within the empirical personalities whose central organs the *buddhis* are as if it were happening within themselves. The *Puruṣa's* failure to distinguish between himself and the *buddhi*, including the whole empirical personality with its mental and sensory activities, is called ignorance (*avidyā*) and is the cause of bondage, for the *Puruṣa*, to the round of births and deaths undergone by the empirical personality.

Unlike classical Sāṅkhya which asserts the essential difference between Nature (*Prakṛti*) and an infinite number of Spirits (*Puruṣas*) and is therefore a pluralistic dualism, the Advaita Vedānta of Śankara postulates the essential oneness of reality in all its aspects—material, mental as well as spiritual—and ascribes to all individual things and beings a common ground or essence which is called *Brahman* and whose nature is one of pure existence, pure consciousness and pure bliss (*sat-cit-ānanda*), three concepts which, to the intellect, appear to be the separate constituents or qualities of some underlying substance, but which in Śankara's conception form a unity of the spiritual essence of reality itself. Advaita Vedānta is therefore an idealistic monism.

Man as an individual is also of the same nature. In essence

he is a spirit (*Ātman*) that is entirely identical with *Brahman*. *Ātman* within the individual—just as *Brahman* within reality as a whole—is the deepest and purest kernel of the personality and, from the superficial, empirical level, he remains unapproachable, unperceivable, even unthinkable and outside the categories of space and time. He is simply inaccessible to the ordinary subject-object type of experience.

What then, is man's empirical self? For, obviously, man does experience himself or his own existence every moment of his waking life and Śankara does not deny it. What man experiences as himself, however, is not his true and pure self (*Ātman*), but his limited empirical self (*jīvātman* or *jīva*). The nature of the empirical self is explained by two metaphors: either as a reflection of the true Self (*Ātman*) in the mirror of ignorance (*avidyā*) or as a limitation or an empirical "dress" (a limiting "adjunct"—*upādhi*) imposed partially on the unlimited Self by ignorance. Ignorance is therefore the creator of the illusory experience of separateness of individual selves from each other as well as from the universal Self, while in reality there is only unity, which is by no means diminished or impeded by the illusory separateness. It is the same as with space, which is also infinite and one, but which nevertheless appears to be split into a multiplicity of enclosed spaces like those in pots or rooms and other enclosed areas. The limitations are there, but they do not really abolish the infinity of space and do not split its oneness into a real plurality of quite separate spaces.

But what gives rise to this ignorance that reflects the true Self in itself as in a mirror, and makes it appear in man's experience to be a limited self, and how do the limitations arise that create the illusion of separately existing individual selves?

The answer to these questions is analogous to that concerning the origin of Īśvara, the Lord, and of the world. In reality only *Brahman* exists, which is the same as to say that only the universal Self (*Ātman*) exists. So it makes sense to ask for an explanation concerning the existence of the limited self only from the point of view of this limited self on the phenomenal, empirical level. To try to project the problem onto the absolute level and answer it there conceptually is a futile attempt. But from the phenomenal point of view it can be said that the universal

*Ātman* enters the empirical person as its self (*jīvātman*) when the empirical person develops during the cosmic process of the emanation of the world.

The empirical person is a complex structure of which the self (*jīvātman*) is the kernel. Various constituents of the structure of the personality form, as it were, layers or sheaths round the kernel. These layers or sheaths correspond to successive stages of consciousness which, in turn, correspond to existential levels or spheres ("worlds"). This is, in fact, an elaboration of the Upaniṣadic teaching on the four states of consciousness. Its formulation was not arrived at by deriving it from the notion of *Ātman* purely speculatively, but—obviously—by a kind of phenomenological analysis of consciousness as it is experienced by the individual in himself.

The starting point of the analysis is the normal waking consciousness on the level of the physical world of objects (*jāgarita sthāna*). What corresponds to it within the subjective experience of the individual is his awareness of his physical body with which he practically identifies himself. The physical body is the grossest sheath of the self (*annamayakośa* or "sheath made of food") called usually the gross body (*sthūla śarīra*). Man's identifying himself with the gross body is a result of his being absorbed in those purely material aspects of life which occur through the body's sense organs. It is the state in which the self has entirely forgotten itself.

The next stage of consciousness is illustrated by the dream experience (*svapna sthāna*). During dreams the gross body with its sense organs is forgotten and man experiences, more easily, the subtler sheaths of his personality—which may also be traced in the waking state, but are usually so overlaid by awareness of the gross body that they are often ascribed to it as its functions. On the basis of the dream experience it is easily possible to see that the function of perceiving and feeling alive is not a bodily process. All those perceptions which in the waking state are furnished by the senses of the gross body, including the feeling of being alive, are experienced equally in the dream state without any bodily awareness and while the bodily senses are not functioning. In the dream state the self is free from the gross body and lives in its double, called subtle body (*sūkṣma śarīra*) or also "character body" (*liṅga śarīra*), which consists of three progressively subtler sheaths of the self: the sheath made of vital force (*prāṇamayakośa*) experienced as awareness of being alive, the sheath made of mind (*manomayakośa*) which is experienced as awareness of mental processes (ideation and thinking) and the sheath made of intelligence or awareness itself (*vijñānamaya-kośa*) which one experiences as understanding.

Thus it appears that the subtle body is what we would call the mental constituents of the personality. The aspect of vitality or awareness of being alive corresponds to the sphere of feeling, whether it is a feeling of well-being, ill-being or neither. The mind (*manas*) includes the mental processes associated with the senses, namely perceptions, ideas and thought, and the faculty or capacity of understanding is that higher mental state which enables a person to see a meaning behind perceptions, ideas and thoughts, and which is different from, although closely connected with, these processes. It is variously interpreted even in Vedāntic literature as intellect, reason or even intuition (and called, as a faculty, *buddhi*). *Manas*. using the material furnished by the physical senses, provides specific thought material, and *buddhi* brings in discrimination, judgment, meaningfulness and actual "knowing". However, all this, including knowing, remains within the phenomenal subject-object world whose basis is the fundamental ignorance (*avidyā*) of the essential oneness.

The subtle body is believed to survive the death of the gross body and to live for some time in corresponding surroundings in the subtle sphere of existence, before a new incarnation takes place.

The third stage of consciousness which is still accessible to, and can, in a way, be known by, an ordinary man, is that of deep sleep (*suṣupti*). In the Vedāntic view deep sleep is experienced as an undifferentiated awareness of bliss (*ānanda*) and it represents the last sheath of the self (*jīvātman*), namely the one made of bliss (*ānandamayakośa*) which corresponds to the "volitional" body (*kāraṇa śarīra*).[1] Bliss is in fact one of the three essential

1. This is usually translated literally as "causal body" which, I think, is misleading. *Kāraṇa* means also motivation, reason, generative cause and volition. The sense "volition" is to be preferred here, as *kāraṇa śarīra* is the bearer of karmic factors from life to life in the process of transmigration, karmic factors being produced by the volitional activities of beings.

constituents of the *Brahman* in itself which is a unity of pure existence, pure consciousness and pure bliss (*sat-cit-ānanda*). But since neither pure lucid consciousness nor purity of being is realized in deep sleep, the experience of bliss during it is not ultimate. Volitional tendencies are still present, albeit dormant, and therefore karmic activities start again when empirical consciousness reappears. Because waking consciousness is split into a subject-object awareness, it cannot take in and preserve the higher unified awareness of dreamless sleep which is subject- as well as objectless (=subjectless as well as objectless) and so there is no recollection in waking consciousness of the state of unification with the Absolute. What remains when one wakes up from dreamless sleep is perhaps a faint and vague aftertaste of a forgotten blissful experience.

The empirical consciousness also remains unaware of the "volitional body" (*kāraṇa śarīra*) which is the sum total of man's karmic actions that accompanies *jīvātman* into future rebirths. The real Self (*Ātman*) which is without limitations is realized only when the fourth (*turīya*) state of consciousness is achieved (as described already in the *Māṇḍūkya Upaniṣad*) which in Vedānta is called (*samādhi*) and described as the individual's pure experience of the ultimate oneness. As such it points to the next chapter.

## Chapter IV

# INDIAN CONCEPTIONS OF SALVATION OR FINAL FREEDOM

The concept of salvation, deliverance or final freedom has been the dominant motive for philosophising in India from at least the time of the Upaniṣads till the present day. But as a matter of fact, all systems of philosophy anywhere in the world tend to strive, in one way or another, to reach some form of absolute or final solution to the problem of existence in general and man's existence in particular. Not even materialistic philosophy is an exception to this, for the following reasons:

Firstly, a materialistic philosopher views reality with the eyes of one who believes that he has discovered the real nature of existence which, for him, is material; therefore he is convinced that during his life he can handle, shape, and change it according to his aims, provided he learns the laws of nature and can apply his knowledge. Secondly, he believes that the final solution of the riddle of existence will come about for him as an individual when he dies: he will be no more. This certainly is one possible conception of final freedom: release from a limited form of existence, because that is what existence as an individual is felt to be. And in the vision of the materialist it is abolished after death by absolute and final nothingness or non-existence.

Whatever this final nothingness or non-existence or the idea thereof may really represent, it has been cherished as a valuable final solution to the problem of existence by some important philosophers, such as Epicurus. And in spite of a superficial fear of death and subsequent non-existence, the idea of finally coming to rest for ever does correspond to a certain basic longing of the human heart to find eternal peace. This desire is often expressed even in Christian prayers for deceased ones and in inscriptions on tombs. Eternal peace or eternal rest, rather than eternal life in heavenly bliss, seems thus to be a more desirable outcome of man's vicissitudinous life.

Desirable and satisfactory as such a solution—on reflection—might be, according to Indian philosophical thinking it is contrary to the nature of things, or to the universal law, to expect to cease to be after death. Nothing can disappear altogether. According to the law of balance things can only change their form. And this is even more true for "living things". Nobody can expect to escape from existence by a mere physical death. The final solution requires much more than waiting till one dies or choosing voluntary death. It has to be sought and pursued with determination and persistence, but finally it can be achieved.

This whole problem was already fully known to some seers of the Vedic times and, obviously, to a part of the general population also. The Vedic hymns show that the normal attitude of men in ancient India was to enjoy this life on earth. The desired life span was a hundred years. After that they hoped to continue living in the heavenly world of fathers and gods. But they already suspected that life after death was not eternal either, and it was uncertain what would come afterwards. So the wish was often expressed in the hymns to attain immortality, in other words to achieve salvation, a final solution to the uncertain situation of man in life and in the afterlife. "Lead us to immortality" (RV 5,55,4)."... may I be released from death, not reft of immortality.." (RV 7,59,12)—this is how the worshipper expresses his anxiety.

There is no indication in the Vedic hymns of what immortality was meant to be like for the individual who would achieve it. We cannot view the often-mentioned immortality of the gods and some fathers living in their company as the final solution, for their immortality was only relative, not a real one. It depended on the availability of the drink of immortality (RV 9,106) and of offerings on earth. And in some Vedic hymns there is another conception of immortality, referred to quite clearly. The best example is the hymn on the creation of the world out of the primeval spirit (*puruṣa*—RV 10,90). One quarter of this cosmic *Puruṣa* was transformed into this world, the remaining three quarters are "immortality" (*amṛta*), in other words transcendence which is beyond manifested existence in time and space. This may well have been the immortality some Vedic sages aspired to.

The Brāhmaṇa texts are not explicit about the final state of one who has overcome repeated death (*punarmṛtyu*). But the aim of gaining freedom from death is pursued persistently, although mostly by means of sacrificial rituals, in agreement with the underlying philosophy of these texts written by generations of priests devoted to their ritualistic practices.

There are, however, indications that the pursuit of immortality by other means than ritualistic practices ran outside the Brāhmanic tradition and was not reflected in the Brāhmaṇa texts, although it was very strong. It prepared the ground for later unorthodox movements like Buddhism and also for the new outlook of the Upaniṣads.

* * *

In the Upaniṣads the situation becomes entirely clear when the teaching on the round of rebirths (*saṁsāra*) is fully grasped in all its implications. The prospect of a never-ending sequence of existences appears to the Upaniṣadic thinker as highly undesirable: however satisfying some lives or some portions of some lives may be, in the long run the constant change of scene, the constant necessity of new births and deaths, is felt to be unbearable and an escape is longed for. Salvation or the idea of immortality takes therefore the form of final liberation from the necessity of being reborn in any place and in any form.

This desire for freedom from existences in limited forms and with limited duration is combined with the illuminating realization that deep down, in the essence of his own personality, man is one with the essence of the universe or with the Divine source of all existence, that the kernel of the individual, his self (*jīvātman*), is the same as the kernel of the universe (*Ātman*) and this in turn is one with the source of existence (*Brahman*).

The final freedom is achieved by one who knows this, assert the Upaniṣads. It cannot be arrived at by good deeds, for they lead only to temporary rewards, nor by ritual actions, for they may only bring one to heaven in company with gods who themselves are "postcreational". It is knowledge alone as a personal, individual achievement which, paradoxically, breaks the shell of individuality and enables the knower to arrive at the realization of the underlying universal oneness.

This liberating knowledge is of an entirely different kind from ordinary knowledge within the world, which is concerned with the objects of this manifested universe. It is also different from knowledge gained from religious texts of the Vedas. Knowledge in the ordinary sense implies a knower or a subject of knowledge and that which becomes known or an object of knowledge. And, as later philosophical investigation adds, there is a third element involved in ordinary knowledge, namely the act of knowing. But the liberating knowledge of the Upaniṣads is beyond the duality of the knower and the known, and the third element, the process of knowing as a process, is absent, too. "You cannot see the seer of seeing, you cannot hear the hearer of hearing, you cannot think the thinker of thinking, you cannot know the knower of knowing." (Bṛh. Up. 3, 4, 2).

The Upaniṣads struggle with words to express this paradoxical fact that the *Brahman* or *Ātman*, the highest reality, is unknowable, and yet it is only when it is known that freedom is won.

But in their own way, the Upaniṣads make the problem quite clear. Knowing *Brahman* conceptually amounts to not knowing it or knowing it only in a very limited way "If you think: 'I know it well', you know but little : only the limited form of *Brahman*", says the Kena Upaniṣad.[1] When Yājñavalkya, the great sage of the Bṛhadāraṇyaka Upaniṣad, tries to give some idea of what *Brahman* is, he carefully avoids giving any idea of it whatsoever and employs negative terms explaining that *Brahman* is nothing that can be described in words or pointed at.[2] Knowing *Brahman* in the real sense means becoming *Brahman* or rather becoming aware that one is and has always been *Brahman*, that one's self (*jīvātman*) is the universal Self (*Ātman*) which is *Brahman*. This knowledge is freedom and freedom is this knowledge. The Kena Upaniṣad puts it this way : "To the knower it is unknown; to the ignorant one it appears known. But he attains immortality who conceives it, having known it through awakening."[3] In other words, those

1. *yadi manyase suvedeti dabhram eva api nūnam tvam vettha brahmaṇo rūpam. Kena Up.* 2, 1.

2. *Brh. Up.* 2, 3, 6; 3, 9, 26: 4, 2, 4; 4, 4, 22; 4, 5, 15.

3. *avijñātam vijānatām vijñātam avijānatām; pratibodha-viditam matam amṛtatvam hi vindate. Kena* 2, 3-4.

who have adequate intellectual knowledge about the requirements for knowing the Ultimate Reality directly (the Yogis under training) are clearly aware of the fact that they do not know it really; those learned theologians or philosophers who believe that they know it, have only a conceptual, second-hand knowledge of it (without being aware of this fact), a knowledge which does not count in the ultimate sense; therefore they can be called ignorant. The real knowledge when the Ultimate is reached, is an intuitive or supraintellectual act of knowing which is not in fact knowing, but an awakening to one's inner essence as the essence of everything. Therefore the resulting knowledge of reality in its totality as well as in all its parts is not a mediated one like knowledge of objects gained through the process of sense perception and its conceptualisation by the mind, but it is a direct experience of everything, including the deepest kernel of oneself and the heart of reality itself, from within.

This deep and penetrating knowledge reveals the essential oneness of all that exists, and of transcendence, without abolishing the surface diversity which, however, no longer obstructs the deep inner vision and resulting freedom.

As we saw in the previous chapter, the experience of oneness is accessible to everyone during deep sleep when the individual consciousness is united with the inner self and, consequently, with the Universal Self. But as the nature of everyday consciousness is rooted in the duality of subject and object, it cannot retain or take in this deep experience of unity and recall it afterwards as a memory. Therefore deep sleep appears to man's surface consciousness as a state without any consciousness. It is only when knowledge through awakening is attained that the continuity of consciousness is retained even during the experience of the individual's unification with the absolute. That is then the fourth state (*caturtha* or *turīya*) which is given the description, among others, of "the essence of the experience of one Self".[1] This experience of the fourth state of consciousness is the result of meditation or Yoga effort (as shown in Maitrī Up. 4, 19 and 7, 11).

1. *eka-ātma-pratyaya-sāra...Māṇḍ. Up.* 7.

But what happens to the personality of one who has acquired the liberating knowledge? He is, of course, liberated from everything that would be experienced as limitation. First of all he is liberated from desires. This is possible, because there is nothing left that he could desire. When he realizes himself as the essence of the world, he possesses everything in a way which is infinitely superior to any form of worldly possessions (Bṛh. Up. 3, 5; 4, 4). Externally he therefore prefers to possess nothing and he lives as a wandering mendicant (Bṛh. Up. 4, 4, 22), unfettered by, and unattached to, anything. Further, he does not suffer, he is free from all evil. No evil can harm him any longer and he is therefore free from any sort of fear. His works (*karma*) can no more reach him in the form of reward or retribution. Whether they are good or bad, they get burnt on liberation as grass does in fire (Bṛh. Up. 4, 4, 22; Chând. Up. 8, 4, 1; 4, 14, 3). His future deeds will produce no karmic effects for him, either. Naturally, he will do some actions as long as he lives, but having become one with the Universal, he has no particular interests any longer and will therefore act as one who does not desire anything for himself and who possesses and applies the highest knowledge when acting (Bṛh. Up. 4, 4, 23).

The attitude of the Upaniṣad, namely that the liberating knowledge with all its effects can already be gained during one's lifetime, is quite in line with the oldest tradition of liberated *munis* as confirmed even by the Ṛg Veda (RV 10, 136). Apart from this tradition, however, there is another one, supported by numerous instances in the Upaniṣads, to the effect that full immortality and liberation, the final unification with the *Brahman*, is achieved only in the moment in which the wise one dies.

Both these conceptions have survived throughout centuries till the present day, not only within the Hindu tradition, but also in Buddhism, although in a doctrinally modified form. The expectation of salvation after death has been more widely held by religiously minded followers of spiritual teachings. The ideal of liberation during one's lifetime has usually been the aim of those who aspire for spiritual leadership and become teachers of others.

The Upaniṣadic teachings on salvation are a result of various trends in the development of ancient Indian religious and philosophical thinking, both within and without the Vedic tradition. Various movements outside the official Brāhmanic tradition were very strong in the time of the early Upaniṣads and one of them became prominent even to the extent of endangering the continuation of the Vedic tradition as represented by the contemporary Brāhmanic system. This movement was Buddhism. It did not finally succeed in replacing Brāhmanism, but managed to reduce its influence considerably, at least for a time, not only among the educated élite of the country, but also in the broad masses of the population. After the strong impact of early Buddhism subsided, Brāhmanism regrouped its position and regained its strength, changing its character in the process quite substantially, so that it was thereafter called by a different name, viz. Hinduism. The further development of Buddhism and Hinduism then proceeded side by side for more than a thousand years in mutual polemics, both movements influencing each other.

* * *

Early Buddhism has a great deal in common with the teachings of the Upaniṣads—as we have seen in previous chapters. Salvation or final freedom in Buddhism is, as in the Upaniṣads, liberation from the round of births and deaths (*saṁsāra*). It is also a situation in which the liberated one is free from all desires. No indication is given in the scriptures of early Buddhism as to the positive contents of the state of liberation. The technical term used for the final achievement is *Nirvāṇa* (Pāli: *nibbāna*) which is mostly interpreted as "going out" or "blowing out" (like a fire or flame). The most favoured definition of *Nirvāṇa* in the texts is "extinction of thirst" (or of craving—*tanhā*) or—a bit more explicitly—"extinction of desire, hate and delusion" (*lobha, doṣa, moha*), elements of the human personality which are characterised as the "three roots of evil".

The Buddha's attitude in teaching was highly pragmatic. He concentrated on making his disciples do their best to achieve *Nirvāṇa* rather than to spend time trying to understand rationally what *Nirvāṇa* meant. Therefore he consistently refused to answer questions pertaining to problems of transcendence that were not yet accessible to the experience of the questioner. Instead he always pointed out what steps the questioner should take to develop his own vision so that he could see *Nirvāṇa*, for himself.

Yet when we do what the Buddha perhaps would not approve of, and examine his instructions and his encouragement of practices that lead to *Nirvāṇa*, we are able to find some indications of the direction in which a conceptual circumlocution or periphrasis of *Nirvāṇa* may be sought.

First of all, *Nirvāṇa* is undoubtedly a transcendental state, for it is not accessible to current human knowledge based on sense perceptions and the deliberations of the mind, nor is it a part of the reality around us and it is not reality as a whole, either. Reality as a whole is, for early Buddhism, just *saṁsāra*, the sum total of all possible experiences of existence in all existential spheres of the universe. *Nirvāṇa* is nowhere to be found within, or in connection with, the structure of the universe.

At the same time, however—and this is the second point of this attempted periphrasis of *Nirvāṇa*—*Nirvāṇa* has to be viewed as immanent. Not being a part of the edifice of objective reality or this edifice itself and being therefore inaccessible to any form of objective scrutiny, it is notwithstanding said to be experienced by one who has won it. Therefore it is immanent or inherent to living experience. But this living experience is not readily available to every individual. It emerges within a man's mind only when his mentality has undergone a complete transformation. The personality, hitherto incapable of direct profound experience unconnected with the functioning of senses and conceptual thinking, has to acquire, in the process of mind training, higher faculties of direct perception or vision, bypassing the ordinary senses and intellect. First this vision extends to other dimensions of existence than that of our material world, both lower and higher, and it may reach such perfection that the meditator is able to perceive with his inner eye (called by the texts usually "celestial eye,'—*dibba cakkhu*) all the subdivisions of *saṁsāra*. He is also able to recollect the innumerable lives which he has gone through from beginningless times and in all possible existential spheres. In this way, in his retrospective vision, he experiences saṁsāric reality in its totality from within, as it were. From beginningless times he has been roaming through variegated existences and experienced everything which can be experienced within *saṁsāra.* While he retains this memory, the future cannot bring him anything new. Prepared by this global experience, the mind of the meditator is then able to dissociate itself from further involvement in saṁsāric experience, to transcend it and to attain to a direct knowledge of *Nirvāṇa* beyond *saṁsāra*.

When the saṁsāric planes and normal means of cognition have been transcended, the direct experience of *Nirvāṇa* cannot be classified as objective or external. It is internal to the experiencing mind and therefore immanent. In this way *Nirvāṇa* can be paraphrased as an experience of transcendence in immanence.

A liberated person in Buddhism is no more an ordinary man. He has become either a *Buddha* (Awakened One), if he has attained liberation on his own and then teaches the way to it to others, or an *Arahat* (Worthy One), if he has won liberation as a disciple of a Buddha. But what is he in himself, what has become of his personality?

It appears that during the lifetime of a liberated one his phenomenal personality, which is composed of the five constituents described in the previous chapter, continues functioning normally, with one profound change which his experience of *Nirvāṇa* brings about in the fourth constituent, the "bundle" of volitional processes (*saṅkhāra khandha*): he has no personal motivations whatsoever. Life in its usual form as a pursuit of satisfactions through personal and social achievements has no meaning and fascination for him, but it is not repulsive, either. So there is no reason for him to go on living as a limited person in limited surroundings. But neither has he any reason to make an end to his life, because the personal and circumstantial limitations do not touch him any longer. He is beyond their reach. Consequently he does nothing to influence the natural course of his phenomenal life process and just waits for it to come to its normal end when the bodily organism is worn out and dies.

Under special circumstances a liberated Buddhist may resort to what others would call suicide, for example if his body is gravely ill and is a nuisance both to himself and others, requiring to be looked after. This would be a waste of time in a community of monks whose prime concern should be to meditate. Such suicides of *Arahats*—approved of, or at least tolerated, by the Buddha—are reported by the Pāli Canon (e.g. MN 144).

But while an *Arahat* is alive, he leads a restrained, quiet life, mostly as a monk, although several *Arahats* were reported who were lay followers of the Buddha and carried on with their worldly duties. In the course of his training towards the attainment of *Nirvāṇa* a traveller on the Buddhist path develops many unselfish tendencies in his character in order to counteract the natural instincts and personal motivations on which a man normally lives and which are always self-centred even if they are sometimes or often socially acceptable or even useful. These unselfish tendencies, such as friendliness to and compassion for others, continue to have effect on his outer personality even after he has overcome all desires. They, in fact, remain in him as the only motivations for any activity. He then assists others in so far as they may be dependent on him for their welfare—if he lives in the world—but primarily he helps others towards a better understanding of life, its suffering and the way to solve it; in short he promotes knowledge of the Buddha's teaching.

In the case of a Buddha, these tendencies are developed to a degree which is described in the texts in terms of a cosmic vocation. Every Buddha is a world teacher. In the distant past he had taken a decision not only to achieve liberation for himself, but to teach others the path to liberation, and he had been training himself for the task during many incarnations. As a result when he gains liberation he also attains the perfect wisdom of an Enlightened One together with all "magic" powers enabling him to be a perfect individual teacher to everybody who approaches him for instruction.

But with respect to the attainment of *Nirvāṇa* itself, whether one is an *Arahat* or a Buddha, this achievement is experienced as final. It is, in either case, total freedom from compulsion of any kind and there is nothing more to be done in this whole universe. After death there is no automatic rebirth, for its driving force, the thirst to live, has completely disappeared. The functioning of the five constituents of personality stops altogether and the person in question "cannot be seen by gods and men" any longer (DN 1,45). He has passed beyond the universe or existence as we know it and as we can imagine it.

But this unqualified situation of a departed liberated one does not mean non-existence as some Western scholars tended to interpret *Nirvāṇa* when they first encountered its descriptions in Pāli sources and as some individuals were also inclined to think of it, even during the Buddha's time. Neither should one imagine that the liberated one exists after death eternally in some way. The Buddha condemned equally both the belief that a liberated one had a permanent existence after death and the belief in his complete annihilation.

The logic of the time accepted four categories of statement about the existence of a person after his final departure from *saṁsāra* : "He is", "he is not", "he is as well as is not" and "he neither is nor is not". The Buddha dismissed all such questions as unprofitable.[1] The dimension of a liberated one who is no more connected with his last body in *saṁsāra* is one which escapes all attempts at conceptual classification.

* * *

Another trend of thought which was partly outside the main stream of orthodox Brāhmanic tradition, but is reflected in some Upaniṣads and later on influenced Hindu thought on a popular level through philosophical portions of the Mahābhārata, particularly the Bhagavad Gītā, developed finally into the classical Sāṅkhya system of philosophy. Its legendary originator is said to have been the sage Kapila who is believed to have lived in the seventh century B. C. The earliest literary account of Sāṅkhya available nowadays is the "*Sāṅkhya Kārikā*" by Iśvara Kṛṣṇa,

1. *Some Sayings of the Buddha*, pp. 292-4; 302-3.
Important works dealing with the problem of *Nirvāṇa* are :
R. Johansson : *The Psychology of Nirvana*, London 1969.
G. D. Welbon : *The Buddhist Nirvāṇa and its Western Interpreters*, Chicago and London 1968.
H. Hecker : *Das buddhistische Nirvana*, Hamburg 1971.

probably from the third century A. D. Sāṅkhya is now recognised as one of the six orthodox systems of Hindu thought.

As we have seen earlier, Sāṅkhya conceives the human personality as a structure created by *Prakṛti* (nature) for the *Puruṣa*, who identifies himself with it because of his ignorance of his true spiritual character. As a result of this illusion the *Puruṣa* suffers all the vicissitudes of saṁsāric life. Liberation can therefore be acquired by him through discriminatory knowledge (*viveka*) which removes that illusion.

As all cognitive organs are parts of the phenomenal personality structure and, consequently, products of *Prakṛti*, it means that training towards the discriminatory knowledge goes on within the prakṛtic processes themselves. *Prakṛti* indeed cooperates, according to Sāṅkhya, for the sake of the liberation of the *Puruṣa*. The process of developing right discriminatory knowledge is a process of purging *buddhi* or intelligence—which is basically sattvic in character—of rajasic and tamasic elements (i. e. elements of energy experienced as passion and of inertia experienced as sluggishness). When *buddhi* becomes purified, it acquires the quality of transparency and can reflect the true spiritual nature of the *Puruṣa* who then realizes that he is purely an onlooker (*draṣṭā*) in saṁsāric processes. He is then able to watch uninvolved even his own empirical (phenomenal) personality as an object (*dṛśya*) without identifying himself with it, just as he could formerly watch some other objects in this world, if he was indifferent to them.

From that moment on the *Puruṣa* is free and *Prakṛti* stops functioning for him. His empirical personality continues living as long as the momentum of the body lasts without his being involved. He is during that time a living liberated one (*jīvanmukta*). After the death of the body he enjoys full freedom without a body (*videhamukti*). *Prakṛti*, of course, continues operating for other *Puruṣas* who are not yet liberated. The free *Puruṣas* can continue to watch the world process without ever being in danger of getting involved again and being deluded into participation. They exist in eternal purity and free from all activity.[1]

The classical form of Sāṅkhya philosophy has never become widely held and is of little influence nowadays, but popularised

1. Cf. A Sen Gupta : *The Evolution of the Samkhya School of Thought*, pp 48-50.

Sāṅkhya conceptions abound in the voluminous Indian national epos Mahābhārata and also crept into the Purāṇas. But the uncompromising Sāṅkhya pluralism of the classical treatises is resolved in popular Sāṅkhya usually in the sense of the empirical plurality and transcendental unity of the *Puruṣa* which is also viewed as Īśvara (the Lord) or the highest God.

* * *

The main tenet of the Upaniṣadic teachings, namely the essential unity of individual beings and the world with their common source (*jīvātman = Ātman = Brahman*) gave rise, in the course of centuries, to the classical system of Advaita Vedānta (nondualistic final teaching of the Veda) which has become most known and influential through Śankara's presentation.

Liberation in Śankara's interpretation is the realization of one's essential identity with the Ultimate Reality called *Brahman.* As in almost all other Indian systems of thought, it also means in the Vedānta system freedom from the necessity to transmigrate from life to life, and freedom from all limitations of phenomenal existence within this universe which is bound by time and space and which, from the position of the Ultimate Reality, appears to be unreal.

But Advaita Vedānta stresses more than any other Indian system the positive contents of the experience of liberation. When ignorance is removed and a man no longer identifies himself with his limited and transitory phenomenal personality, in other words, when he realizes his true nature which is the same as that of the world and of its source, the *Brahman*, he acquires in fullness and purity what he experienced in the phenomenal world only imperfectly and in a lessened or subdued way or only occasionally, namely existence, consciousness and bliss (*sat-cit-ānanda*).

However preferable, during a man's life, existence appears to be to death, it is a miserable and shadowy existence compared with the pure and full existence of a liberated one, an existence which is beyond the limitations of space and time. However clear man's consciousness may be at times, it appears very faint and limited in the light of pure and free consciousness after liberation. And whatever pleasurable experiences man may have in the phenomenal world, they are always mixed with sorrow of some kind and are too brief; but the pure bliss experienced by a liberated one has no limitations whatsoever.

Advaita Vedānta also equates liberation with perfect knowledge. Liberation according to it is not a result of knowledge, knowledge itself is liberation. To use the often discussed comparison: when one sees a snake, there is fear. But when one suddenly realizes that what one thought to be a snake was, in reality, only a piece of rope, the fear is gone. The knowledge of the real nature of the coiled object is liberation from fear.

The liberating knowledge can be attained already during one's lifetime. But if obstructions to knowledge are too strong, they may prevent it from maturing fully during one's lifetime so that some adepts are fully liberated on physical death only. Śankara accepts both possibilities, liberation during lifetime and liberation on bodily death (*jīvanmukti* and *videhamukti*).

A *jīvanmukta*, one liberated during his lifetime, becomes entirely free from any possible fruits of his previous *karma* that have not yet started manifesting themselves. (The technical term for this unmanifest karmic load is ***sañcita karma***). During the rest of his life he does not produce *karma* for the future (*āgāmi karma*), because he does not act as an individual for individual aims, which is possible only when one is ignorant. But those past karmic seeds which have already started having effect (*prārabdha karma*) cannot be stopped and have to come to full maturity. The *jīvanmukta*, however, accepts them and remains balanced and unaffected by them, no matter whether they are good or bad. He lives in full knowledge of his true essence, and events on the phenomenal level, although not unreal in themselves, do not reach the depth of existence in which he is centred.

So there is actually little difference between a *jīvanmukta* and a *videhamukta*. Existence in the body being no more a burden or a limitation for a liberated one, its disappearance on death does not mean much to him. His worldly personality disappears and he is no more traceable on the phenomenal level, but the world itself does not disappear and he can still remain in touch with it, if he so wishes. But his view of it is completely changed and shifted from the surface of things into the underlying essence, the Ultimateness. Thus he remains forever unperturbed by the world and its events as the depth of the sea remains unmoved by the waves on its surface.

Although Śankara's interpretation of final liberation has been the most influential one within the development of Hindu thought, it has by no means been universally accepted, the chief objection against it being this: that it does not leave any space for the individual when he reaches liberation; he just merges with the absolute *Ātman* and does not exist any more. But the Upaniṣads are not so explicit on the subject and allow other interpretations of the final situation than that of a strict transcendental monism. And so the Vedānta philosophy developed two other main lines of thought which are represented by Rāmānuja (12th century A.D.) and Madhva (13th century A.D.), although they have never become as famous as Śankara.

Rāmānuja's teaching is known as "qualified non-dualism" (*Viśiṣṭa-Advaita*). The Highest Reality, the *Brahman*, is for Rāmānuja also the highest God who has existed from eternity. His nature is spiritual, but he has also a body. Before creation this body was a subtle one and the creation of the world is actually a transformation of God's subtle body into a grosser one. Individual beings are also a part of the creation. They are different from each other—they are beings in their own right—but they all together form, in conjunction with the material things of the world, the *Brahman's* body. They have, of course, a higher status than things. An individual, while being himself, is, at the same time, *Brahman's* attribute. He can realize his true nature by gaining final knowledge and salvation, which does not mean the end of his existence as an individual, but opens for him a life of permanent intuition of God without ever having to undergo a transformation into the state of creation again.

Madhva's interpretation of *Vedānta* asserts an absolute plurality of selves that are entirely different from, but entirely dependent on, *Brahman*, the Supreme God. In the state of liberation which, according to Madhva, cannot be achieved without the will and help of God, the self, the individual, continues existing as such, having become free from bondage to the world and from any form of suffering. He lives delighting in eternal adoration and worship of God.

* * *

An important development of the conception of final liberation took place within the Mahāyāna school of Buddhism which started during the first century B.C., if not earlier. The goal of traditional Buddhism was the achievement of Arahatship by the individual follower of the Buddha's teaching who thus won for himself the final freedom known as *Nirvāṇa*, while the world and other beings in it continued their saṁsāric existence. The new movement stresses the limitations and dangers of this outlook. In concentrating on one's own salvation one may develop a narrow-minded and selfish attitude and completely miss the goal which, in fact, is the transcending of the prison of individuality. Therefore the formulation of the goal of the new teaching is broadened. The Mahāyānist does not want to follow the historical Buddha and win his personal salvation as the Buddha's disciple. He rather aspires to go in the footsteps of all previous Buddhas, men who not only reached final freedom, but also acquired perfect enlightenment and became teachers of mankind.

This is an elaboration of the philosophy of liberation which has not been open to Hindu thought, where salvation is mostly understood as obtainable on the basis of knowledge inspired by the Divine source. Hence the idea of teachers of mankind has taken there a more traditional religious form than in Buddhism and is represented by the mythology of divine incarnations (*Avatāras*).

For a follower of the Mahāyāna ideal of Buddhahood it means a very considerable postponement of his achievement of final freedom. For he renounces entering *Nirvāṇa* to which he may be very near and takes upon himself the *Bodhisattva* vow. A *Bodhisattva* is one who struggles through innumerable lives to develop qualities called perfections (*pāramitās*) which constitute a Buddha. When he finally reaches the state of perfection, he becomes a Buddha of a certain period in history and teaches the liberating doctrine of Enlightenment to others. At the end of this last life of a world teacher he passes into the final *Nirvāṇa*.

In this form the new teaching does not appear to be basically different from the traditional one, it simply gathers round itself those individuals who want to serve a broader purpose in the cosmic context of producing Buddhas for future world periods. However, soon the conception of *Nirvāṇa* and Buddhahood itself began to be reformulated and elaborated beyond the conceptual grasp of the traditional Buddhism.

Firstly, we find in the Mahāyāna scriptures the puzzling statement that *Nirvāṇa* and *saṁsāra* are not different from each other. *Saṁsāra* is *Nirvāṇa* and *Nirvāṇa* is *saṁsāra*. A liberated one has not acquired anything and has not passed to any other place from where he has always been. Secondly, the idea that Buddhahood might be a state of mind to be created in a person or developed in his mind is refused. If Buddhahood, the perfect enlightenment, were something to be produced or grown by the unenlightened person, nobody would ever have a chance to become enlightened. How could perfection be developed by someone who is totally imperfect and has so far had nothing to do with it ? If Buddhahood is obtainable, it is only because one is already in possession of it. Buddhahood is the true nature of everything and everybody. The task is to realize or to uncover it fully without stopping half-way as, according to the Mahāyāna view, the *Arahats* do.

A third point concerns the status of the Buddha as an historical personality or of Buddhas in history in general. It is no longer seen necessary to aim at becoming a Buddha in a certain historical period. The realization of Buddhahood within oneself is what really matters.

Strange as these new formulations may sound when contrasted with the traditional teachings of early Buddhism, they really only reformulate in new and positive terms what, by implication or in germ, was already contained in the early teachings. The new formulations were prompted by the increasingly rigid and unfruitful spirit of the Buddha's followers in most monastic communities within a few centuries after the Buddha's death. In the absence of his inspiring personality the individual follower's concentration on his own spiritual progress often led him into isolation from the community of lay followers and to the loss of reliable criteria of his progress. In his pursuit of the ideal of becoming an *Arahat* who had to overcome all the fetters that tied him to the world, but who did not have to gain the full knowledge of a Buddha, it was possible to mistake cultivated indifference to the world and people around him for the balance of a really freed mind. So the new stress on acquiring full enlightenment and wisdom equal to that of a Buddha, in other words, realizing perfect Buddhahood, was a natural safeguard against possible self-deception on the part of a would-be *Arahat.* In this context it is no wonder that the *Bodhisattva* path was considered superior to the path of a mere follower of the historical teachings of the Buddha.

While pursuing his ideal of Buddhahood, a *Bodhisattva* is not a follower of the historical Buddha and his teaching as preserved in the words and written texts of the Canon.[1] What a *Bodhisattva* is doing is re-discovering step by step the truth (*Dharma*) itself. Therefore he is able to reformulate it ever afresh and does not have to cling rigidly to inherited texts. But although the form of presenting the truth to others may be different from the wording of the traditional teaching, the spirit remains the same.

The primary aim of a *Bodhisattva* is to assist other beings to obtain or to get nearer to liberation. For the sake of this aim he renounces everything that would gain an advantage only to him. He does not want anything for himself, not even *Nirvāṇa.* Even when his spiritual maturity brings him to the threshold of *Nirvāṇa* and it would require only a little step to crown his efforts as an individual truth-seeker by achieving *Nirvāṇa,* he turns back from it to stay in *saṁsāra* for the sake of helping others. Paradoxically, this very step of turning away from *Nirvāṇa* secures it for him in a far superior way. For staying in *saṁsāra* in order to serve is an act of supreme renunciation, the highest possible expression of perfect selflessness. And perfect dissociation from the self and self-centredness is what *Nirvāṇa* is about. The *Bodhisattva* therefore finds himself in *Nirvāṇa* while at the same time he has stayed and continued active in *saṁsāra.*

It is the constant process of appropriating bits of *saṁsāra* for oneself that makes one remain tied to *saṁsāra* and blind to the fact that *Nirvāṇa* is here and now. Appropriation means limitation and perpetuation of the prison of saṁsāric personality. But

1. This is so despite the fiction maintained in many Mahāyāna Sūtras to the effect that the historical Buddha actually preached the new doctrine outlined in them under unusual circumstances, e.g. to gods and other supernatural beings.

when self-centredness is abandoned and the narrow personal vision of happiness and freedom is broadened by compassion for other suffering beings and replaced by selfless struggle to free others, the chains of personality are broken and it is then no more a prison for a limited mind, but a vehicle for an enlightened mind to help the world. An accomplished *Bodhisattva* is entirely free and enlightened while remaining active within *saṁsāra* into which he keeps being reborn. He renounces the final *Nirvāṇa* of a Buddha, whatever that may be, until all suffering beings are released, that is until universal liberation is brought about.[1]

* * *

The idea of a liberated one who does not withdraw from the world process—either into a transcendental *Nirvāṇa* or into a Divine element—but remains active within it, who not only is no more subject to its limitations but is virtually working on its improvement and final spiritualisation, was a new development in Indian thought. As mentioned earlier, it was not an idea that corresponded to the usual Hindu attitude to the question of universal salvation. Yet it was too appealing a vision to remain entirely confined to the Buddhist Mahāyāna perspective and has gradually exercised a deep influence on Hindu thought as well. It has finally found expression in the philosophy of Śrī Aurobindo Ghosh.

1. The development of Mahāyāna Buddhism has not yet been satisfactorily explored. Nor is there a reliable comprehensive work which would systematically cover this vast field. It may be considered useful to study the following works :

D. T. Suzuki : *Outlines of Mahayana Buddhism*, London 1907.

E. J. Thomas : *The History of Buddhist Thought*, London 1933.

Har Dayal : *The Bodhisattva Doctrine in Buddhist Sanskrit Literature*, London 1932 (repr. Delhi 1970).

E. Conze : *Buddhism. Its Essence and Development*, Oxford 1961.

,, *Buddhist Thought in India*, London 1962.

A. K. Warder : *Indian Buddhism*, Delhi 1970.

E. Lamotte : *Histoire du Buddhisme Indien*, Louvain 1958.

According to Aurobindo's philosophical outlook, individual salvation is a small achievement, especially if it is enjoyed in seclusion or isolation from the rest of a creation left behind by the liberated one. The true salvation to be aimed at includes the salvation or spiritualisation of the whole cosmos. Therefore a man who strives after liberation should be preparing himself to become a tool of universal salvation. His preparation takes the form of the spiritual integration of all the constituents of his being with the Divine Supermind. That means that the whole of his personality has to be spiritualised: his mentality, including his intellectual capacity, his lifeforce or vitality—with all its biological instincts—and also his material body. Nothing is abandoned or thrown away in the final integration. The process of spiritual growth is not one of elimination, but one of transformation.

An integrated individual who has reached salvation has achieved it not only by getting to know himself in the deeper layers of his mind, that is by reaching perfect self-knowledge which is always an important part of every spiritual training, but also—and more importantly—by opening his mind to the Divine Supermind which lifts him to the status of a Superman or Gnostic Being. This status is above any sense of individuality in terms of self-centredness or self-interest. The consciousness of a Superman is infinite, his mental faculties are unlimited and he has a great power for illuminating others and spiritualising his environment. But he does not altogether cease to be an individual, for he will still use a body and will be appearing in the world. His body will not, however, be an autonomous product of Nature, but as an integrated part of his personality as a Gnostic Being, will function under the full control of the Supermind with which the Superman is one. On the level of the Divine there is no contradiction between the individual and the universal or between the personal and the impersonal. Both are inseparable aspects of one and the same reality.

Having accomplished the integration and spiritualisation of his own personality, Aurobindo's Superman directs his attention to assisting other people towards the same—or perhaps it is better to say towards a similar achievement, for although there is oneness within the Divine, there is no actual sameness among individual Supermen. At the same time the Superman exercises a spiritualising influence on all his surrondings: on nature and on society and their various processes. In the long run, with more Supermen active in the world, the whole world will be spiritualised. A further stage will include the spiritualisation of the entire cosmos.

Although this outline of Aurobindo's vision might indicate that the final transformation of the cosmos is bound to come in any case—as a result of a long-term evolution under the influence of the Supermind, it is not so. The Divine mind will not act, unless there is a receptacle prepared for it. And the preparation of the receptacles rests with the efforts of individuals. Unless there is at least one integrated individual who has developed his mind and purified his personality to the point of having transcended his individuality, the Supermind will not start working. And only if others follow suit, and also achieve the status of Supermen so that an élite of spiritual beings will appear in the world, can the process of spiritualisation of the earth and subsequently of the whole cosmos be set going under the influence of the Supermind.

The Supermind is prepared to descend and work through developed individuals whenever one or more of them reaches the necessary status (although this process must not be viewed as an automatic one). But if in a culture at a certain stage of evolution which requires for its preservation and further growth a Divine intervention, the Divine power on descent does not find prepared receptacles, that is if there are no individuals who have worked sufficiently for their salvation, it cannot descend and revitalise that culture, with tragic consequences.[1]

Śrī Aurobindo's philosophy thus not only presents an individual searching for freedom with the prospect of a high achievement

1. There seems to be some evidence that Aurobindo thought of himself as influencing the affairs of the world as a channel for the forces of the Supermind. See A. Marshall : *Hunting the Guru in India*, London 1963, pp. 61-63.

in becoming a Superman, but confronts him, at the same time, with a high responsibility for triggering off, or at least contributing to, the final liberation of the whole cosmos.[1]

1. The source of Aurobindo's views is his main work "*The Life Divine*" and other voluminous works, all published in Pondicherry. There are several shorter expositions describing his philosophical teachings e.g.: *The Integral Philosophy of Sri Aurobindo. A Commemorative Symposium.* Ed. by H. Chaudhuri and F. Spiegelberg, London 1960.
"Sri Aurobindo", a chapter of the book : R.S. Srivastava : *Contemporary Indian Philosophy*, Delhi 1965, pp. 109-155.

## CHAPTER V

# YOGA, ITS ORIGIN, PURPOSE AND RELATION TO PHILOSOPHY

Any attempt at an explanation or definition of Yoga necessarily involves going into the questions of its origin and purpose and its relation to the development of man's philosophical thought and also his religious ideas and experiences. The country of origin of Yoga is undoubtedly India, where for many hundreds of years it has been a part of man's activities directed towards higher spiritual achievements. Yet when we want to find a clear definition or a general description of Yoga, the Indian texts do not help us directly. To describe Yoga, even in Indian terms, requires research into its past history and present situation.

The question of the origin of Yoga can be looked at from two different angles. Firstly, there is the problem of its historical origin in the distant past in India. And secondly, we may feel that it is also important to inquire into the psychological reason for the appearance of Yoga. On this point if we can say that there are features in the human psyche that suggest that there is also a psychological explanation for the origin of Yoga, the question then arises whether what is known as Yoga is a purely Indian phenomenon or whether equivalent or similar developments can be found elsewhere in the world and if so, what is peculiar to Indian Yoga when compared with those other developments.

But wherever we start, a preliminary description of Yoga is unavoidable. Broadly speaking, Yoga is the conscious and directed activity of an individual aspiring to a suprasensory and supraintellectual experience which is to him of spiritual value and which fully or to some extent transforms or deepens his life and his knowledge or understanding of reality and of himself. This obviously means that the aim of Yoga is to bring about a higher or more accomplished state of mind which transcends man's usual everyday experience and opens for him a new field of vision and the capacity to grasp this vision. The whole personality becomes transformed and can function in a new dimension hitherto unknown or inaccessible to it. Knowledge is widened, deepened and increased and there is a sense of communion with the infinite or with the essence of all things or with reality as a whole. This experience is extremely satisfying and fulfilling and often uncovers for the individual a source of inspiration which makes his life creative and enables him to assist or lead others.

When described in this way, Yoga cannot be viewed as having been confined to India. There is obviously a psychological force in man which compels him to strive for fulfilment through transcending himself. Perhaps this force can be described as manifesting itself predominantly in three forms.

Firstly there is the longing of the human heart to escape from, or to overcome, its loneliness. Man becomes aware of his loneliness when he discovers that he is an individual. As long as he feels safe in his parental home, his neighbourhood, his social class, his political party or his tribal community, this problem does not arise. But in practically all conditions some individuals discover the astonishing fact of being on their own. Man as a self-conscious individual separated from the environment and facing other individuals he knows only from outside, feels extremely lonely and this state of lonelinessis unbearable to him. He has to find a link to some other individual or to some other entity and form a relation that will enable him to escape, at least to some extent, the boundaries of his individuality. For a time—which may be very brief or last a lifetime—this aim may be fulfilled in a relationship of love with a partner or children or both. Sometimes it is some kind of vocation that covers the loneliness—social work, work for one's country or even revolutionary activities.

But all the experiences and satisfactions such relationships and activities can give, do not really abolish the solitude and self-enclosedness of the human heart, they only cover it up or obscure it temporarily. Therefore some individuals try to break out of the prison of individuality into the wider realm of a transcendental spiritual reality in which they feel at one with the essence of reality or with reality as a whole or with the Creator.

This is the domain of magic, ecstatic practices, mysticism and also, of Yoga. In direct experience a link to, or identity with, a higher and deeper world dimension is established in which the individual is no longer cut off from the whole.

Secondly, there are occasional experiences in perhaps everybody's life that might be described as temporarily opening a channel in the individual to a wider and deeper dimension of life than the one to which the individual normally has access. When an attempt is made to describe the nature of these experiences, the words "intuition" and "inspiration" are used. Some individuals can resort to this source of direct communication with reality "from inside" more often than others. The forms in which they express these experiences—if they do so at all—may be different: artistic, religious or philosophical. A frequent source of inspirational experience is also man's communication with nature, when its beauty, majesty, peacefulness or creativity impresses his mind. Under favourable conditions several elements of inspirational and intuitional value may combine to create a climate of higher achievement and closer relatedness to the universal in which the individual may feel entirely fulfilled. The Taoist movement in China at one time produced such a climate. When such intuitional experiences are inspired by or occur within a religious tradition, a whole mystical movement may appear, such as Sufism within Islam.

However, the experience of intuitional contact with a deeper dimension of reality, which mere sense perception and thinking cannot achieve, is not confined to artists and mystics, but also plays a substantial part in scientific discoveries. If progress in scientific knowledge were a result of nothing but collecting data about reality and then thinking about them and systematically describing them, this progress would be steady, regular and even predictable, because there are always hard-working scientists doing just that. But the chief scientific discoveries have been made by scientists who besides their knowledge of the relevant facts and their capacity to think logically, also had ideas which could not be logically derived from generally known facts and from the accumulated data in their field of research. These ideas often occurred to them when they were not engaged in their actual work, but were quietly musing or even resting. Then a moment of inspiration allowed them to see into the "heart of the problem" and make a new discovery. If this kind of intuitional contact with the heart or essence of things as distinct from a mere sensory and conceptual encounter with them could be methodically cultivated, science and human knowledge would benefit enormously. This is the idea that was at the cradle of phenomenology. Husserl's "viewing of the essence" (*Wesenschau*) is or aims to be the mind's direct contact with the heart of things which is made possible when their sensorily perceived qualities and conceptually defined character are abstracted ("bracketed out").

Thirdly, there is the incessant and insatiable urge inherent in the human mind to seek more and more knowledge about the world and about itself which occasionally turns into a pursuit of wisdom, of a global view or experience of reality or of "truth as such". This pursuit may remain a conceptual one as most systems of philosophy show, but sometimes it overflows into a burning desire to penetrate the whole truth fully, to solve the mystery of existence directly in one's own heart, but, at the same time, with a degree of validity which could be called universal.

One example of this development in European philosophy is Plotinus. In India philosophy reached this stage several times and each time either Yoga played an important part in it or philosophy came very near to what Yoga strove for.

If Yoga in this broad sense of the word has not been confined to India, and the equivalents of Yoga have existed in other countries as well, what, then, is specific about Indian Yoga and why has it such an appeal for people in other parts of the present-day world, particularly in the countries with a Western civilisation whose scientific achievements have conquered the world and imposed its way of life all over the earth and therefore also on India herself? Why are some men of science and some philosophers and even some prominent personalities of the Christian religion studying Yoga and sometimes trying to experiment with it or to utilise it in a practical way in their respective fields?

The answer to these questions is threefold: Yoga shows some affinities with Western scientific methods, it appeals to some trends in European philosophical thinking and, besides, it promises to help revive the practically dried up tradition of Christian mysticism or at least of living piety.

All this can be said about Yoga because it is the only form of mystical or spiritual practice that has survived for several thousand years, has not remained, or has never been entirely, affiliated to one particular philosophy or religious creed, and has developed some specific and independent methods of inquiry and practice which can stand critical examination and are applicable also in modern conditions of scientific scepticism. The pursuit of spiritual experiences that Yoga claims to make possible does not necessarily presuppose an individual's previous commitment to any particular philosophical or religious faith or tenet. The sole requirement for Yoga practice is a spirit of inquiry that does not stop when the limits of conceptual research and analysis are reached and the method of "direct seeing" or "viewing" is to be learned and systematically applied.

There is a spirit of discovery about Yoga that is similar to that often found in modern scientific research. In this field of activity of the human mind Yoga also shares with science the characterstic of a methodical and systematic approach to its task.[1]

With regard to philosophy, the initial chapter could provide some conclusions that point towards the possibility of resorting to Yoga methods, or of deriving help from them when the philoso-

1. The literature in which Yoga and Western scientific investigation are confronted or brought together is not yet very numerous, although it is steadily growing. Apart from some physiological observations it is mostly psychology, psychotherapy and psychiatry which show interest in Yoga and seem to be able to benefit to some extent from the encounter. Some highly interesting material has been gathered in the book : *Forms and Techniques of Altruistic and Spiritual Growth. A Symposium*. Ed. by P.A. Sorokin, Boston 1954.

Another important Symposium on the subject was held by the Stuttgart association "Arzt und Seelsorger" : *Abendländische Therapie und östliche Weisheit. Ein Tagungsbericht*. Ed. by Prof. W. Ritter. Stuttgart 1968.

Individual scientists and therapists have also engaged in the study of Indian Yoga and sometimes its practical utilisation. The best known of them is C.G. Jung and of the more recent ones E. Fromm is noteworthy. The following two books are also of considerable interest:

H. Jacobs : *Western Psychotherapy and Hindu Sadhana*, London 1961 (rewritten in German by the author as *Indische Weisheit und westliche Psychotherapie*. München 1965.

M. Boss : *A Psychiatrist Discovers India*. London 1965.

phical quest has reached its utmost limit in conceptual analysis. One could also speculate whether certain elements of the Yoga approach might not be found useful or interesting by some exponents of phenomenology, since the affinity of Yoga with the phenomenological method seems so clear. And further, there is a whole new field of research called Comparative Philosophy that concerns itself, among other things, with investigating interpretations of Yoga experiences.[1]

The idea of Yoga helping Christians to become better Christians is no longer a novelty. The appeal that Yoga has had for wide circles of people in Western countries has not escaped the attention of Christian organisations and individuals interested in enriching their own religious life. Both the physical and meditational techniques of some schools of Yoga have been found methodically helpful in initiating and heightening or intensifying the mood of piety and religious experience in believing Christians who otherwise were not easily able to find similar help from within their own tradition.[2]

To summarise : the uniqueness of Yoga and its great value for our time lie in the fact that it is based on a living tradition that has remained efficient since ancient times; that it has developed systematic methods for pursuing and reaching its aim; and that these methods can be applied and studied today both on the popular level by people with personal inclinations towards following a spiritual path and on the academic level by research workers in various fields such as comparative religion, the history of religions, philosophy, psychology, psychotherapy and physiology. All other forms of mystical practice are, by contrast, largely a matter of the more or less distant past (e. g. the ancient Greek mysteries, Egyptian magic practices, Gnosticism, various

1. Abundant material for pursuing this question can be found in the volumes of the magazine "*Philosophy East and West*" published by the University of Hawaii.

2. See J. Herbert : *Yoga, Christianisme et Civilisation*, Lyon 1951. Other French authors writing on the subject are : J.M. Dechanet and Fr. Lambert. Important are the works of the German Roman Catholic priest Hugo M. Enomiya-Lassalle S.J. :

*Zen—Weg zur Erleuchtung*, Wien 1960.

*Zen-Buddhismus*, Köln 1966.

*Erleuchtung des Zen-Buddhismus und Christliche Mystik* (a contribution to the Stuttgart Symposium mentioned above).

forms of shamanism, and mediaeval Christian mysticism) or if they are partly alive, which some might claim to be the case at least with Christian mysticism and Islamic Sufism, they are closed systems accessible only to believers. To be sure, there are movements within Yoga which also are closed systems, such as those which can be joined only by converts to a particular sectarian belief or by followers who have acquired faith in one particular Guru, and there are also secret traditions into which a newcomer can be initiated only after long preparation. But there is plenty of scope for a critical approach and for scientific research in Yoga. Some present-day Yogis do not object to scientific experiments being carried out on them when they practise their exercises or meditation, and there are methods of Yoga training available to any research worker ready to put them to the test by taking them up personally.

Progress in all research work is, naturally, slow and this is even more true of research in Yoga. The novelty of the subject and the requirement of personal involvement in Yoga training present difficulties to the Western way of research that have hardly been known before, because the scientific approach has been based mostly on external observation and laboratory methods of experimentation. These methods may be applied, with some success, to certain aspects of Yoga, but they cannot lead very far, for Yoga's "laboratory" is the mind—and in advanced stages it must be just the experimenter's own mind. That is why the popular demand for some form of Yoga practice in the West has overtaken the cautious and slow advances of academic research. As a consequence the popularisation of Yoga and its practice in the West is in the hands either of Eastern gurus with little or no understanding of the Western psyche and tradition or of Western amateurs with varying degrees of competence.

Under these circumstances it is all the more necessary for Yoga to be studied and experimental research into it to be conducted on all possible levels and from all angles.

The historical origin of Yoga in India belongs to the distant past, and when and how it began cannot be established.[1] Some

1. The subsequent pages are based on my paper "Religious Practice and Yoga in the Time of the Vedas, Upaniṣads and Early Buddhism"

scholars of Indology and Comparative Religion (such as H. Oldenburg, J. W. Hauer, J. Gonda, M. Eliade) expressed the opinion that Yoga developed in connection with or as a result of religious practice in the Vedic and post-Vedic times and on the basis of primitive or archaic shamanist and ecstatic practices surviving parallel to the official religious worship of Brāhmanism. It is their contention that whatever elements of what later became known as Yoga can be traced in the ancient Vedic worship or in the unorthodox magic practices of the so-called *Vrātyas*, they were only the preliminary stages of specific forms of Yoga that developed later. Thus, in their view, Yoga virtually established itself only some centuries after the Vedic period, reaching its peak in the classical Yoga system of Patañjali.

This, we may say, is an evolutionary view of the origin of Yoga, based on the nineteenth century evolutionistic thinking that has largely dominated Western historical research. According to this conception the human mind has developed from primitive stages of understanding that were mythological and magical and basically confused to more realistic stages of knowledge based on a more or less conceptual understanding of the world which includes grasping abstract formulations of various laws, such as that of causality, and which leads to systematic

read at the Symposium, *Aspects of Religion in South Asia*, organised by the School of Oriental and African Studies, University of London, 30th March—2nd April 1971. The paper was published in the "Annals of the Bhandarkar Oriental Research Institute", vol. LVI, Poona 1975, pp. 179-194.

The main works quoted in the paper are the following :

J.W. Hauer: *Die Anfänge der Yoga-Praxis im alten Indien*, Stuttgart 1922.
" *Das Vrātya. Untersuchungen über die nicht-brahmanische Religion Alt-Indiens*, Stuttgart 1927.
" *Der Yoga. Ein indischer Weg zum Selbst*, Stuttgart 1958.
H. Oldenberg : *Die Religion des Veda*, Stuttgart 1917.
M. Eliade : *Yoga, Immortality and Freedom*, London 1958.
J. Gonda : *Die Religionen Indiens I, Veda und älterer Hinduismus*, Stuttgart 1960.
V.G. Rahurkar : *The Seers of the Ṛg Veda*, Poona 1964.
H.D. Griswold : *The Religion of the Ṛg Veda*, London 1923.
A. Ch. Bose : *Hymns from the Vedas*, London 1966.
H. D. Sharma : *Contributions to the History of Brahmanical Asceticism*, Poona 1959,
R. Choudhary : *Vrātyas in Ancient India*, Varanasi 1964.

and conceptual formulations of Man's knowledge and to the elaboration of exact methods of acquiring it.

It may well be accepted that man's mind has passed through different stages of conceiving and expressing its experience of life and reality and that the present stage can be described as conceptual, intellectual or, perhaps, scientific, while in India three or four thousand years ago it was not conceptual and could be called mythological. But any claim that our knowledge and understanding of life and reality are higher, because we conceptualise them, cannot be maintained. Science has brought vastly improved technology and consequent mass production of material goods, but the problems of life, its frustrations and aspirations, have remained the same, and man's ability to cope with them seems, if anything, to have been diminished rather than increased by his technological advances.

According to the Indian tradition, the ancient Vedic religion is not a product of the imagination of primitive minds reacting to natural phenomena by personifying, worshipping and dreading them, but on the contrary is the creation of exceptional individuals who had reached the fullness of mystical vision, which gave them an understanding of and insight into the problems of life and existence that may have amounted to the final knowledge of the truth itself. As we have tried to point out before (chapter II), the way in which those individuals passed on some portions of their knowledge to the people was determined by the idiom of the time, which was not one of concepts, but one of imagery and religious magic rites.

There is no reason why the Indian claim should be rejected and the Western evolutionary theory imposed on the history of Indian spiritual endeavours—or, for that matter, on the history of religions in general. When we examine the known spiritual or religious movements, we find that there have always been one or more spiritually advanced individuals at the beginning of these movements. It was only later that there followed a period of formalisation in which elaborate worship, ritual and formulated faith played an important role, and still later came conceptual elaboration of the doctrine, and possibly dry scholasticism. Later still, a kind of revival of the original mystical vision may have occurred once or a number of times, but at no later stage in the history of a religious tradition can it ever be viewed as spiritually higher than it was at its foundation, and certainly a conceptual elaboration of an old spiritual teaching cannot be considered a higher stage of development.

When Yoga is looked at in this light, it must be said that the admired and no doubt admirable exposition of Yoga by Patañjali gains nothing, on account of its conceptual and systematic form, over the previous Yoga sources. In fact, the freshness of the expression of deep spiritual experience in some Upaniṣads may even point to or indicate a more immediate contact with the transcendent on the part of their authors than, we might feel, is indicated by the succinctness of Patañjali's Sūtras. Likewise when we compare the Buddha's exposition of his Eightfold Path with Patañjali's Eightfold Yoga, we have to admit that although Patañjali's is the more systematic of the two, his Sūtras do not clearly lead many people to believe—as the Buddha's sermons obviously do in the case of many of his followers and admirers—that there is a profound knowledge of truth itself and full enlightenment underlying them. And some hymns of the Ṛg Veda and Atharva Veda, if studied carefully, lead us to admit that only deep experience based on efficient Yoga techniques could have produced the profound insights that we find in them despite their language, which often seems very alien to us in its imagery, symbology and enigmatic quality.

It follows therefore that the idea that there can be something like an evolution in Yoga (and, by the same token, in mysticism of any kind), as far as its essential achievements are concerned, cannot be upheld. There are changes only in the form of transmitting the Yoga experience, changes in description and interpretation and in the exposition of what can be called the path to the Yoga accomplishment. These changes are perhaps responsible for the appeal which Indian Yoga has for Westerners. Through these changes its descriptions became comprehensive, and to the Western mind they make it appear as if Yoga itself had undergone "evolution", for some of the Yoga expositions form a successive line, as it were, from mythological and symbolical texts to conceptual and systematic expositions, a pattern so familiar to European thinking.

From what has been said so far it follows that it is not really proper to speak about a historical origin of Yoga. What is perhaps possible is to try to trace historical sources of information about the occurrence of Yogis and Yoga practice in the past in India, as far as historical research permits us to do so.

The very earliest indication—though not a proof, strictly speaking—of the existence of some form of Yoga practice in India comes from the pre-Vedic Harappan culture which can be dated at least as far back as 2700 B.C. A number of excavated seals show pictures of a figure seated in a Yoga position that has been used by the Indian Yogis for meditation till the present day. One of the depicted figures bears signs of divinity (which reappear in later centuries on pictures of the Hindu god Śiva, himself worshipped as the Lord of Yoga by some sectarian Yogis), others are without them, being apparently human. The position of the figures is important. Many seals found in Mohenjo-daro and Harappa picture scenes from religious life and mythological events which obviously were of great significance to the people of the time. The seated deity and other figures, undoubtedly absorbed in meditation, indicate that mental Yoga exercises were known and played a substantial part in the religious—or can we perhaps even say philosophical—outlook of the epoch.

Another seal shows a figure sitting cross-legged—with rearing cobras in front of it. Thus all the three aspects of yogism that are well known from later centuries as well as from present-day India are indicated on the seals: the Yogis who emphasise the human character of Yoga endeavours, the Yogis who belong to some religious tradition and worship their *Īśvara* (Lord), and those who belong to a popular trend that is marginal to Yoga and is best designated as fakirism. Archaeological discoveries allow us therefore to speculate with some justification that a wide range of Yoga activities was already known to the ancient people of pre-Āryan India. Understandably, nothing definite can be said about the ideological or theoretical background of these activities.

The situation is a little less difficult in Vedic India, but it is by no means easy to draw a picture of the state of Yoga practice and knowledge of that time. Even when we accept sympathetically the view that the Vedic literature which is the sole source of our knowledge originated with inspired or enlightened seers, the form in which it has been preserved bears unmistakable signs of much lesser minds who were at work when the hymns were arranged into collections of four Vedas. This work was done in the age when orthodox priesthood became a very important force in society and the predominant religious practice was ritualistic and highly formalised. There was little understanding among the priests of the deep mystical vision of the individual seers of old. They had a stereotyped world view based on the primary importance they attached to ritual sacrifices, and they arranged the Vedas to suit their ritualistic needs. Many important hymns were thus obviously lost because they were excluded from the collections, and others were changed by the redactors so that their original meaning became somewhat obscured.

However, there are references in many Vedic hymns to what on closer analysis appear to be hints at or descriptions of Yoga practices and achievements. Quite often they are found also in hymns describing sacrificial rites and this led some scholars to believe that Yoga practices developed from or as a by-product of religious observances. But this assumption is wrong, for other hymns give evidence of Yogis who were independent of the religion of the time. They roamed the country and their sole objective was to reach transcendence and live in touch with it. The presence of Yoga elements in religious rites shows, on the contrary, that there was a considerable influence exercised by Yoga on the religious practice of the time.

The most striking evidence of the existence of advanced Yogis outside orthodox religious circles is furnished by the *Keśin* hymn (RV 10,136). This hymn apparently does not belong to the category of inspired pieces composed by ancient *ṛṣis* (seers), but makes the impression of having been written by someone who did not himself belong to the loose fraternity of the "long-haired ones" (that is what the expression *keśin* means). He was perhaps a sympathetic observer, broad-minded enough to record the phenomenon, but not sufficiently experienced himself to understand it so fully as to give a clearer account of it than he did.

The long-haired one is described in the hymn as someone who is on friendly terms with the natural elements and is equally at home in this world as in the spiritual world, is a master of the creative flame present in himself and is at one with the light of wisdom. He travels around homeless, clad only in dust (or, perhaps, in a yellow robe of rags). His is the path of the winds, he is inscrutable to other people, a companion to gods, belonging, in fact, to another dimension of life. Others can see only his body; his mind or real personality dwells in the "inner region", in the centre from which he can see everything that has taken form and understand the whole world. Gods are his friends, he is one with life itself, dwelling simultaneously in the physical and spiritual universe. He is seen as a gentle friend not only by gods and other higher beings, but by all other creatures, including wild beasts, and he knows what is going on in the hearts of all other beings he encounters. He has mastered all the forces of the universe, even the dark ones, and unharmed endures and overcomes all the vicissitudes and dangers of existence.[1]

The culture of ancient India was not as unitary as it appeared to the first European students of the Vedas. As already indicated, the Vedas in the form in which they have been pre-

1. For a discussion of some points raised by the *Keśin* hymn and the views of previous scholars refer to my paper quoted above. A detailed analysis of the hymn has recently been given by J. Miller in her article "Forerunners of Yoga : The *Keśin* Hymn" published in the book, *A Reappraisal of Yoga*, London 1971 (in co-authorship with G. Feuerstein), pp. 94-120. Her interpretation presents a fresh look at the problem of Yoga in Vedic times and is imaginative and bold. Yet she does not go as far as drawing the final conclusion that the *Keśin* hymn portrays an accomplished Yogi (although the title of her article—Forerunners of Yoga—might indicate it). But this step has to be taken, if one does not want to subscribe to the unfounded positivistic evolutionary theory of the development of Indian religiosity from primitive to "advanced" stages, of which Yoga would also be a result or by-product. The view that the top Yoga achievements had already been reached in ancient times and nothing substantial was added to them later on does not exclude acceptance of the finding that Yoga techniques underwent systematisation in subsequent centuries and there is no doubt that descriptions of Yoga practice and achievements developed from mythological accounts to conceptual systematic expositions.

served do not reflect the real nature and different trends of the ancient Indian civilisation, but present it through the medium of the Brāhmanic conception. The Brāhmans (priests) endeavoured to create a unitary cultic civilisation based on their religious leadership, and to a great degree, although not entirely, they achieved this goal for a time, and also retrospectively, by eliminating most sources of non-Brāhmanic tradition and brahmanising the rest.

But for several centuries during the second millennium B. C., and possibly also for one or two centuries of the first millennium B. C. as well, there were two distinct centres or areas of civilisation in Northern India. One, which can be called the Vedic civilisation proper, was in the west, reaching as far to the east as the rivers Jamuna and Ganges, and the other was further east, with its centre in Magadha. The latter was the territory of the so-called Vrātyas. The society there did not develop a class of priests as happened in the Vedic area in the west. Instead they preserved for a long time an ancient mysterious institution of semi-military religious brotherhoods that gradually produced, in conditions of partly settled life which was becoming more settled, an aristocratic class and rulers (*rājanyas*) over the settled part of the population on the one hand and small religious communities practising magic on the other. These were then the Vrātyas proper. Their name probably means "those who have taken a vow" and indicates the religious nature of their communities. Some groups of Vrātyas were almost constantly on the move and performed various rites for settled folk. They also often visited the western Vedic area for the same reason and were in high esteem with the people there because of their reputation as magicians. But the Brāhmans looked down upon them as barbarians, for undoubtedly they were undesirable rivals for them.

Some Vrātyas also lived as solitary wandering ascetics and had a reputation for holiness. They were no doubt another example of ancient Yogis. Even the group practices of small teams of Vrātyas contained elements of Yoga practice, particularly of the kind later known as Tāntric Yoga. The Vrātyas also certainly produced an extensive literature of their own, but it has not been preserved as such. A part of it has survived in

Brāhmanic redaction in the Atharva Veda, for as the process of brahmanisation of the ancient Indian culture continued, the Vedic culture also spread to the east and gradually absorbed the Vrātya culture. However, a substream of non-Brāhmanic trends in religion, yoga, and philosophy remained alive and erupted on the surface a few centuries later. Its bearers in the interim period were anonymous ascetic wanderers, and philosophically-minded aristocrats (*rājanyas*).

The Brāhmanic culture was by then very ritualistic and spiritually sterile and was hostile to the other-worldly and ascetic outlook of Yogis, who generally disregarded ritualistic practice as it did not lead to higher spiritual achievements. It did not, however, remain altogether unaffected by the assimilation of the Vrātya culture, nor by the continuous, although perhaps slender, thread of Yoga tradition within its own Vedic sphere of thought. The Brāhmans, however narrow-minded some of them may have been, could not entirely ignore the Yoga tradition. They could not change, let alone eradicate, the high esteem in which the wandering ascetics were held by other classes of the population, their deep influence on the minds of people because of their magic lore, and their authority over educated individuals interested in metaphysical questions concerning transcendence. As a result Brāhmanism in its aspiration to become universal was forced to include the ideal of the ascetic and Yogic way of life—which was one of renouncing all home and worldly cares, obligations and aims and concentrating on the search for final truth—in its newly elaborated scheme of four stages of life (*āśramas*) through which every Āryan should progressively pass during his life.

In the first stage the Āryan boy became a student of the Divine lore (a *Brahmacārin*) and learned, by heart, such portions of the Vedas as he would later in life need when performing his religious duties. This period of apprenticeship lasted for twelve years and was spent in the teacher's house. At the end of this time the young man's primary duty on returning home was to marry and raise a family. Thus he entered and lived in the second stage of life, that of a householder (*gṛhastha*). When his children became grown-up and themselves in turn married and had small children, it was time for the householder to retire, to go to a forest and live there as a hermit (*vānaprastha*), although he often shared his solitude with his wife. This was the time when, released from worldly duties, he could start pondering and meditating on the deeper meaning of the sacred texts he had once, as a youngster, learned by heart and, as a grown-up member of the community, had then recited in his capacity as head of his family, or, perhaps, even as a professional priest, during his daily rituals (or during sacrificial ceremonies performed for others) which may often have been repeated more or less habitually aud thoughtlessly.

In this way he could slowly penetrate the symbolical and hidden meaning of the texts and of the ritual actions that pointed to the mysterious forces underlying life and the visible universe. When he felt that he had loosened his ties to the world of things and events and could "follow the path of the winds" without being attached to or haunted by past memories, he left his hermitage, this time alone, and became a homeless wanderer (***parivrājaka, saṅnyāsin*** **or** ***bhikṣu***), prepared to leave this world when his hour came, without leaving a trace behind. He thus prepared himself for the final step into the Unknown.

In theory this scheme appears to be ideal, as it offers man the best of both worlds. In practice, however, it was followed by only a few. The bulk of the population, including the priests, subscribed to the idea only theoretically and did not care to embark on the third let alone the fourth stage. On the other hand, zealous young enthusiasts of whatever caste sometimes left home as youngsters, never to return, and pursued the path of Yoga in some way or another for the rest of their lives. There were among the hermits some teachers who became famous for their wisdom and spiritual achievements, and some students stayed with them for life or for as long as they felt they needed in order to absorb their teaching and technique in Yoga with a view to achieving the experience of breaking through to the transcendent. Some of them then in turn became teachers and masters.

On the whole, however, profound spiritual activity existed only as a substream or sidestream alongside the official orthodoxy of Brāhmanism throughout the period of the Brāhmaṇas, and it erupted into the open only in the time of the Upaniṣads (around 600 B.C.), culminating a little later in the appearance of Buddhism along with other non-Brāhmanic movements of which the most important was Jainism.

But the Upaniṣads were not, of course, primarily mystical texts and, as far as the oldest ones are concerned, Yoga figures prominently in only one or two of them. Substantial parts of them are still mythological and religious and their most important portions are philosophical. Philosophical speculation had existed side by side and also been interwoven with the ascetic and Yogic trends since quite early Vedic times, as we have seen in previous chapters. Philosophy was often inspired by mystical vision. As the Creation hymn puts it: "Seers searching in their hearts with intelligence discovered the connection between being and non-being." (RV 10, 129, 4). Without the inspiration provided by direct vision or some form of intuition, philosophy becomes mere speculation based on sense data and finishes as materialism. Pursued with intelligence, philosophical inquiry based on sense data leads to the establishment of sciences which, however, then also tend to be based on a materialistic outlook and have, moreover, a built-in inability to encounter the transcendent, as the development of sciences in the West sufficiently demonstrates.

In ancient India materialist philosophy never acquired any degree of importance and although outstanding results were achieved in some fields e.g. mathematics, the sciences never reached a position from which to challenge the supremacy of the philosophical approach. The philosophy of the Upaniṣads, which belongs to the time prior to the creation of philosophical systems, was not predominantly speculative, but was obviously inspired to a great degree by mystical experiences in which the Yogic approach played an important part.

The oldest Upaniṣads (such as Bṛhadāraṇyaka, Chāndogya, Taittirīya, Aitareya or Kauṣītakī) do not appear to have been directly related to any of the schools of Yoga of the time, but they were definitely under the influence of Yoga trends. That is shown mainly by the importance of the concept *dhyāna* in them. Chāndogya Upaniṣad has a whole section on *dhyāna* (7, 6, 1,) from which it transpires that it was a notion with which the authors or redactors of the text were not quite familiar, but nevertheless the true nature of *dhyāna* does get across in one passage. We can translate *dhyāna* as "contemplative absorption" or, perhaps, "meditative state of mind" which implies in either case a supraintellectual perception and clear vision of reality. The Upaniṣad says that *dhyāna* transcends the superficial or surface mind (*citta*) and that, in fact, everything exists in *dhyāna*, as it were: the earth, the atmosphere, the heavens, the waters, the mountains, gods and men. What it means is that if one's mind has access to the deep cognitive state of *dhyāna*, one sees everything in its proper place, the mind is at peace, balanced and without conflict. Only small people, says the Upaniṣad, live in conflict and create upheaval around themselves.

This picture of a meditative way of living was elaborated later on in Buddhism (see MN 1, 1) and has remained to this day the ideal of all subsequent Yogic and spiritual endeavours in the East. Zen Buddhist descriptions of an accomplished state of mind (which is "no mind", viewing reality as it presents itself without trying to grasp it in any way) strikes the same note, and so does Krishnamurti's call for an observant, alert mind maintaining constant, intelligent awareness.

However, the language of the older Upaniṣads at their best is philosophical. Theirs was a time of great intellectual search for formulations expressing man's knowledge about himself and the world. The mythological language of previous periods had outlived itself and truth-seekers were groping for new modes of expression. They found them in philosophical concepts that largely replaced symbolical images. Mystical and Yogic experiences were also expressed in this new way and were then speculated about. The highest philosophical achievement of the Upaniṣads is their teaching on the nature of reality, which, as we saw, they called *Brahman*, and on the nature of man, called *Ātman*. In the final analysis these two were found to be identical, but it is hardly possible to regard this achievement as the result of purely speculative work. There obviously lay behind it an inner mystical experience which first found its expression in the famous explanation "I am Brahman". The conceptual elaboration followed. We may well assume that it was Yoga practice (the technique of *dhyāna* meditation) that brought about that overwhelming experience of unity, of feeling at one with the whole universe and its creative essence, which then triggered off the Upaniṣadic philosophical speculations along these lines.

In this respect one can regard Yoga as having assisted at the birth of Indian philosophy. But it also brought about religious revival, as has already been pointed out, and certain types of religious worship became interwoven with Yoga techniques. A whole school or schools of religious Yoga developed in which typical Yoga techniques of meditation and concentration were combined with religious worship and piety, the goal being to reach unity or union with God (Śvetāśvatara Upaniṣad is probably the oldest document of this trend, and other Upaniṣads followed).

On the basis of what has been said so far it should now be possible to formulate the difference between Yoga and philosophy and also perhaps between Yoga and religion and to point out what their mutual relationship is.

At the beginning of this chapter we described what we understand Yoga to be. The most important element in Yoga, it has again to be stressed, is its practical concern to prepare the individual for acquiring a direct experience of reality, a kind of supraintellectual vision equal to a reliable direct knowledge of truth itself. Philosophy, on the other hand, although it also aims at arriving at a true knowledge of reality, has no means of achieving this aim in direct perception, because it uses concepts as its medium of knowing. It works through reasoning, speculation and conceptual analysis. Clearly, reasoning, speculation and conceptual analysis are not, in themselves, independent means of gaining new knowledge about reality. The material for them must be furnished by some primary channel of cognition, which is sense perception. The intellect then uses this material—the sense data—to create a more or less orderly picture of the world expressed in concepts. In the course of further reasoning and speculation the intellect also forms complex pictures and theories about those parts of reality that it has not yet got to know with the help of sense perception. Man then tries to verify these more advanced pictures and theories by further investigation of available additional sense data and finds them sometimes wrong and sometimes correct.

Then, at a certain stage of his knowledge of the world and himself, man starts creating complex metaphysical theories about the last principles of reality or about reality as a whole. He tries to circumscribe conceptually the "final truth" which, in fact, as a mere philosopher he can never hope to get to know with certainty by the means at his disposal. But in his efforts he not only utilises the previously accumulated human knowledge now available to him, which he works through thoroughly, using his capacity for systemisation, but also quite often makes use of intuitional (supraintellectual) processes going on in his mind which are sometimes called inspiration. This is a point at which speculative philosophy virtually transcends itself and touches upon a province which cannot be rationally explained or intellectually grasped. Artists, mystics and, of course, Yogis are more familiar with it. And Indian Yoga claims to have elaborated systematic methods of mind training that can be grasped rationally and put into practice which bring the mind eventually to a point that is the threshold of the vast and mysterious sphere of transcendence. Here there is no sense perception, nor does the process of thinking continue. Yet the mind remains alert, awake and perceiving. It is claimed that it perceives reality or truth directly. In other words the mind becomes one with truth.

Inspiration, as it is usually understood, or moments of intuitional insight, are not currently the results of any sort of systematic training; they seem to occur sporadically with some gifted individuals. According to their special interests such individuals then utilise these moments for creating works of art or for some other purpose. If they are philosophers, their philosophising receives an inspirational impetus. The influence of such inspirational moments may be traced in the works of some philosophers, both ancient and modern, and some were well aware of them. Plato, for example, described the state of inspiration in his Phaedrus, and Plotinus elaborated his whole system of philosophy as a result of four brief moments of spiritual vision which he happened to experience during his life. The philosophy of Hegel bears some signs of having been inspired by something more than mere conceptual analysis, and Husserl's phenomenology is, in fact, an attempt to get hold of inspiration or intuitional vision as a regular channel to reality in order to utilise it systematically for enlarging man's knowledge. This aim bears a strong resemblance to the purpose of Yoga.

If an individual who is occasionally visited by inspiration or intuition is a strongly developed religious personality, he may become a prophet, a religious leader or the founder of a new religious movement. If he is a devout follower of an existing religious tradition whose spiritual message he intuitively grasps, he becomes a mystic within that tradition. In the Indian tradition the best example of mysticism is the Hindu movement called Bhaktism, which also produced a systematised path, known as Bhakti Yoga, which utilises the achievements of previous Yoga schools.

It may now be evident how closely philosophy, religion, mysticism and Yoga are related and it is therefore not surprising that confusion as to the nature of Yoga and its relation to religion and philosophy, and whether it is actually distinct from them, easily arises and is, moreover, perpetuated in the minds not only of outsiders, but also of followers of Yoga as is shown by many of the books on Yoga, especially the popular ones.

Of the three disciplines that have just been discussed in relation to Yoga, mysticism is the one nearest to it. Mysticism and Yoga both aim at a suprasensory and suprarational encounter with the transcendent. But while every form of mysticism grew up within a particular religious tradition so that its goal, the transcendent, was defined for it by that tradition, Indian Yoga in its original pure form seems to have been independent of religion and has always avoided defining the transcendent in very definite terms. Of course, mysticism can also reach to these heights of independence: on rare occasions a mystic within one particular religious tradition will attain to such a high vision of the transcendent that he is no longer able to refer to his experience in the language of his religious tradition if he wants to convey some glimpse of it to other people, and then a striking resemblance to some Yogic formulations can be detected in his descriptions. An example of this kind of achievement is Master Eckehart, the mediaeval German mystic.

But as far as we know, only India produced a continuous tradition of independent Yoga, of an uncommitted search for truth without preconceived ideas, which was elaborated systematically and made into a tool for training the mind and the whole personality of man in order to prepare him for the breakthrough into the transcendental realm of freedom.

This tool, this system of training is, of course, available to everybody, including religious believers, and the initial intuitive experiences and limited glimpses of the reality beyond the senses and the intellectual horizon, even if gained with the help of a neutral Yoga training method, may well for some time fit in with their preconceived ideas or beliefs about the Divine. This is even more likely to happen, if—as is often the case—the neutral Yoga methods of training are combined with some form of devotional practice. And so Yoga, in one form or another, can be found throughout the centuries of Indian religious history incorporated in various religious sectarian movements and being used to enhance and deepen their followers' faith and piety, however contradictory the ideas these movements may hold on the surface about the Divine and the final achievement. This is also why, as stated earlier, Yoga methods can be and are being used even by religious circles outside the Indian religious tradition, for example within Christianity. But by the same token Yoga can also be practised by a modern scientific agnostic. If he is open-minded, he may perhaps benefit or gain from it more than religious followers of any kind. In the first place he can find out if Yoga's claim is true, namely whether it really leads to some knowledge beyond the senses and the intellect.

If there is the need or interest, it is always possible to disentangle Yoga and religion, however mixed they may be—in a text or even in a speech. By analysis one can separate statements, descriptions and instructions that are evidently based on a religious belief, on the evidence of some scriptures held sacred by their followers or on an authoritative interpretation by someone who as a Guru requires its acceptance as true or final rather than urging pupils to test and verify his teaching for themselves. For example, if a religious text or an incantation—whether addressing Śiva, Viṣṇu or any other god or directed to a Buddha, all the Buddhas or a Bodhisattva—is recommended for meditation, it is a religious use of Yoga practice. The same holds true for *mantras* with religious significance, for visualisations and for all other exercises. Such instances are plentiful in Yoga texts and schools and with individual teachers. But there is also plenty of evidence in the old Indian texts that entirely neutral methods of Yoga practice were in use in the most ancient times, that they were used throughout the centuries that followed, and can be found in use nowadays.

A modern student of Yoga who wishes to start practising or experimenting with it should therefore be aware of this problem in Yoga and its sources and should find out, first, whether his inclinations allow him or lead him to take up a form of Yoga practice which is linked to or mixed with religious ideas, images and practices. An opportunity to take up Yoga in this way may be the first that will be readily available to him. But quite often the accompanying elements of such a form of Yoga will prove to be entirely alien to his background hitherto. Therefore it may be of greater advantage to search and study a bit more, until he finds a mode of practice that is religiously neutral, rather than try to arouse religious feelings in himself artificially.

The entanglement of Yoga with philosophy is perhaps even greater than with religion, especially because the classical system of Yoga—that of Patañjali—was closely associated with Sāṅkhya philosophy so that historians of Indian philosophy often describe these two systems together. Later on, when Śankara's Vedāntic philosophy became the most influential doctrine in India, many Yogis were its followers and interpreted their practical Yogic experiences in the light of the Vedāntic, often highly speculative, thinking. This tendency still prevails among many Yoga followers in India and has been spread in the West as well, especially by popular authors on Yoga. The expression "Yoga philosophy" that is so often used is quite frequently only another name for a popularised form of the world view elaborated in the system of Advaita Vedānta.[1]

1. The expression "Yoga philosophy" was already used by Vivekananda in his English books. An example of mistaking Vedāntic speculative philosophy for the higher wisdom which supposedly follows when Yoga is mastered is the case of Paul Brunton, for some years a pupil of the late Śrī Ramaṇa Maharṣi of Arunachala who had the reputation of being an accomplished Yogi. Śrī Ramaṇa was not a philosopher, although

But as with religion, it is possible also to distinguish philosophy from genuine Yoga itself. It is of course true that some philosophical elements will always accompany Yoga, but that is no disadvantage just as long as one is aware of them and distinguishes for oneself one's preliminary and accompanying philosophical suppositions from what is the pure content of Yoga experience when some has been achieved. Practically all newcomers to Yoga take it up because they have certain ideas about reality, a certain preliminary world view or even a theory about the world and life and they hope to acquire more certain and complete knowledge through Yoga. Or else they feel that the world as they see it and their life as they live it are not quite satisfactory, that there is something sadly missing in them and they believe that Yoga can open the gate to a new vision of the world for them and will teach them to live a fuller life. This may sound too high-flown a statement and the newcomers themselves might be surprised at it. Nevertheless it does express the underlying attitude even of those who might not be able to express it themselves in a similar way.

This attitude, even when not conceptually formulated let alone elaborated, can also be called a preliminary philosophical outlook, which implies that there is more to the world and to life than is immediately obvious to an average mind. This, perhaps, is the soundest attitude, especially when it is adopted consciously. Although quite a number of Yogis and Yoga followers, in the past and nowadays, have cherished a certain philosophical doctrine, such as Advaita Vedānta, and have been intellectually convinced of its universal validity so that their

in his few short writings he used some traditional, mostly Upaniṣadic, philosophical terms. The reputation of this modern Indian saint was based on his personal influence ("presence") acclaimed by practically all who had the opportunity of visiting him (see e.g. the account given by Baron Dr. Hans-Hasso von Veltheim-Ostrau in *Tagebücher aus Indien* II, Hamburg 1956). However, when Brunton became acquainted with and enchanted by a form of Vedāntic philosophy (through some other teachers and a few literary sources, one of them being Gauḍapāda's *Māṇḍūkya Kārikā*), he thought he had surpassed Śrī Ramaṇa in achievement and dedicated two subsequent books (*The Hidden Teaching Beyond Yoga* and *The Wisdom of the Overself* mentioned earlier) to popularising this philosophy, which he called "mentalism".

Yoga practice has been for them a tool or means whereby they could realise this teaching in their own experience—an attitude not far from that of religious believers—there have always been also truth-seekers who, seeing the inadequacy of human knowledge and the existential situation, set out on a journey of discovery, experimenting earnestly with every available method that might solve the problem of existence, without having to indulge in philosophising about the possible outcome of their search and without feeling compelled to adopt any of the existing philosophical solutions of that problem.

Another point relevant to the problem of the relation between philosophy and Yoga is connected with descriptions and interpretations of Yoga experiences. Again, someone who follows or is inclined to believe in a particular philosophical teaching describes and interprets his partial Yogic experiences in the light of that particular philosophical teaching. Or it can also happen that a philosophical teaching is created in the course of interpreting Yoga experiences. (Two such teachings were reported by the Buddha as being the creations of his two Yoga teachers, Alāra Kālāma and Uddaka Rāmaputta, who both reached certain high Yoga absorptions and interpreted them as the final reality.)

But there are also instances of descriptions that are sober and without an added speculative element. They are then simply accounts of psychological experience during Yoga practice. In the case of Yogis who may be looked upon as having reached accomplishment, the speculative philosophical element can be very conspicuous by its absence. The best example is undoubtedly the Buddha, who—as the earliest Buddhist texts allow us to conclude—never created a systematic philosophical teaching and never attempted to give a picture of the whole of reality in conceptual terms and was always reluctant to describe the final goal of the spiritual path. When he did give some indications of it, he always used non-philosophical terms, trying only to create an assurance in the minds of his followers of the desirability of the final achievement, called Nirvāṇa.

The conclusion resulting from our inquiry in this chapter is this: that careful analysis always makes it possible to sort out the philosophical, religious and vaguely mystical elements from the practical, systematic and psychologically descriptive genuine Yoga elements, if it is desired to do so. It is therefore possible to study, and benefit from, the vast literature on Yoga from whatever school it comes and to experiment with it or to follow its methodical instructions without premature commitment to any particular religious creed or philosophical view.

## Chapter VI

# SCHOOLS OF YOGA

When Yoga is dealt with, it is often done in a way which creates the impression that it is a coherent and unitary system or movement. Inasmuch as our objective is to assess Yoga's value, circumscribe its field and anticipate, in conceptual analysis, its ultimate aim, this way of treating it is unavoidable. But as soon as we try to study the concrete methods and techniques of Yoga practice, we are faced with a variety of approaches, some of which sometimes coexist within various circles of Yogis, while others are exclusive to certain separate Yoga schools. In short, there are a number of types and schools of Yoga and this must have already been so in very ancient times.

On previous pages we have hinted at the possibility, if not quite certainty, of the existence of various types of Yoga as early as in the Harappan culture. The Vedic sources also give grounds for us to conclude that there were various types of Yogis in their time, and the indirect evidence of the oldest Upaniṣads as well as the direct evidence of the Pāli Canon confirm that there were numerous schools of Yoga with different techniques of practice in existence in their time also.

But it is only with Buddhism itself as expounded in the Pāli Canon that we can speak about a systematic and comprehensive or even integral school of Yoga practice, which is thus the first and oldest to have been preserved for us in its entirety. The other systems of Yoga contemporary with early Buddhism are known only from brief references to them in the Pāli sources, but some further evidence of their existence can be derived on the basis of the Upaniṣadic texts and later epic literatures, particularly the Mahābharata. As their tradition has not survived separately till the present time, however, and as no written sources have so far come to light, no systematic reconstruction of the teachings and methods of those schools is possible.

Another school of Yoga that is slightly older even than the Buddhist one and whose system is reasonably well known is Jaina Yoga. But in spite of its greater antiquity with respect to Buddhism, its sources, the Jaina literary documents, were composed several centuries later than the Buddhist ones, and as later developments within the system cannot now be separated from earlier elements, the original form can no longer be reliably distinguished. Therefore the only other ancient system of Yoga comparable with that of Buddhism is the Yoga of Patañjali which appears to be a great synthesis of Yoga trends going back to very ancient times. A part of this process of systematisation and synthetisation leading to the great, although brief, exposition of Patañjali, can be followed in some Upaniṣads. The obvious conclusion is that the different schools of Yoga which may have existed since quite early Vedic times did not develop strong separate identities over a number of generations of their followers, with the result that it was possible for them to be finally absorbed into Patañjali's synthesis without surviving it as independent schools.

## 1. THE YOGA OF EARLY BUDDHISM

As we have already seen, Buddhism was much more than just a school of Yoga. We may say that the teaching of the Buddha aimed, right from the start, at replacing in the minds of its followers both the religion of the day, now usually called Brāhmanism, which was a form of ritualistic worship based on the Vedic tradition, and the current philosophical speculation that was partly reflected in the contemporary Upaniṣads. Both these trends were too cosmos-orientated in their outlook to be compatible with the strictly realistic attitude of a quest for individual liberation "here and now" as expounded in the Pāli Canon.

The story of the Buddha's life itself shows this realistic attitude very clearly. When the future Buddha left home and became a wandering ascetic, he did not join a philosophical school in order to learn the then fashionable art of dialectical discussion, but stayed with various teachers of Yoga as their pupil and subsequently also practised Haṭha Yoga of the prāṇāyāmic variety in the hope of thereby achieving full enlightenment. He later reported that he finally succeeded in his endeavours, after he had perfected his achievements in renunciation and Yoga practice, by deepening his meditations (of the dhyānic variety) and accompanying them by what can be described as heightened awareness and analytical insight.

Subsequently when teaching, the Buddha made use of all his previous experiences, and the resulting set of instructions for spiritual practice was his so-called Noble Eightfold Path (*ariya aṭṭhangika magga*), the first known integral Yoga system.

The form in which the Buddhist path is described in various parts of the Pāli Canon tends to be doctrinal and is obviously intended to meet the needs of the monks, who were homeless full-time followers of the Buddha's teaching and who preserved and finally redacted the Canon, but there is enough evidence in the Canon itself that the path was also followed, already in the Buddha's time, by lay disciples. The form of instruction given to them was bound to be different from that given to the monks, but the Pāli Canon has preserved little, if anything, that would give us a guide to reinterpreting the path in the context of normal living. Yet such an interpretation is certainly legitimate and has been attempted in modern times as part of the presentation of Buddhism to the world at large.

The Buddhist eightfold path is a system of training the mind and the whole human personality for the final achievement of a vision of reality that is far beyond the ordinary capacity of an individual mind to grasp in normal circumstances. Therefore the task of the path is to prepare the individual for the feat of transcending himself. This is done in stages which include unselfish behaviour, impersonal thinking and deep states of meditation in which the individual personality is left behind.

Each of the eight parts of the path, however, has its own stages of development and application—initial and advanced, external and internal, and finally the perfected stages. This means that they do not exactly represent a line of progressive steps on the path to be taken up one by one, but a comprehensive system of self-education and training of all the constituents of the human personality to be attempted more or less simultaneously according to one's capacity, and to be gradually deepened. Only a summary interpretation can be attempted here.

1. *Right viewing* (*sammā diṭṭhi*)

For a follower of the Buddhist teaching as a whole, right viewing may mean looking upon everything in life in the light of the doctrinal formulations so abundant in the Pāli Canon and the commentaries. Such viewing, based on the words of the scriptures, should be gradually replaced by viewing reality according to the spirit of the teaching and finally by directly seeing things "as they really are", as the follower progresses in his individual practice.

However, a modern student of Yoga has to reinterpret the doctrinal formulations to suit his own thinking, keeping in mind, of course, the final aim of Buddhist Yoga. As this is Enlightenment, which implies, among other things, transcending one's own personality, right viewing may be understood as training oneself in viewing individual things, and reality as a whole, in an impersonal or supra-personal way.

The normal attitude of man in daily life is, basically, utilitarian. The objects of the world and other living beings, including other people, that he encounters are, by and large automatically, sorted out according to their usefulness to him. This attitude is more or less instinctual and is illustrated at a tender age: a child shows its interest in things by testing them for their edibility, which it does by putting objects into its mouth. As man grows, his interests multiply, but the attitude remains throughout his life and is expressed in his institutions and in the whole of human civilisation. The Old Testament story of creation sums it up in affirming to us that God created the whole world, with all its natural resources, plant life and animals, to serve man. And our secular modern civilisation is still largely based on this principle: everything is made subject to economic utilisation and quite often even to ruthless exploitation.

Yet there is one feature in modern Western civilisation that comes close to the idea of right viewing, although it has been applied to a limited degree only. This is the idea of objective knowledge, which has so far been best developed in the area of scientific research. (It has its roots in the philosophical inquiries of the ancient Greek philosophers, starting with the sophists and Socrates, but in modern Europe the sciences have revived the spirit of objective inquiry into what is true, while the humanities have only slowly followed with, so far, a somewhat smaller degree of success.)

When a scientist is investigating an object, trying to get to know all about it, he refrains from personal interests, inclinations and idiosyncrasies of all kinds and describes it objectively without emotional comments. Thus an entomologist when dealing with insects will study their bodies, sense organs, degree of intelligence, if any, and pattern of life, and describe his findings in much the same matter-of-fact way whether the the insect in his hand is a beautiful butterfly or an unpleasant bed-bug. If he did not proceed in this way, he would not obtain adequate knowledge about the insects. In the long run, of course, knowledge gained by scientific research is made use of for current human needs, although it may originally have been sought simply because of man's urge to add to the store of human knowledge.

When one is training oneself in right viewing, the approach is nearly the same as during a scientific investigation: one tries to look at things in an impartial way, objectively, without preconceived ideas, prejudices and immediate aims or regard for personal advantage, and without allowing emotional reactions to interfere and divert the mind's attention to the practical or utilitarian aspects of the object encountered. In this way one learns more about things, people, events, the world and the laws that govern them than by following the habitual patterns geared to self-interest, satisfaction and gain. Training in right viewing means learning to look at reality from a higher perspective that transcends man's personal interests and in the long run aims at seeing every single thing in the context of the whole of reality, in other words from the view-point of the Absolute, whatever this may be taken to mean.

2. *Right thinking* (*sammā saṅkappa*)

The doctrinal Buddhist formulation of right thinking is twofold. Firstly it is described as thinking that is free from greed, ill-will and cruelty (e.g. in DN 22) and secondly as thinking turned away from worldly pursuits and preoccupied with the eightfold path and its goal, Enlightenment (e.g.MN 117).

In other words, right thinking follows naturally, if right viewing is practised. Efforts to transcend narrow personal points of view and goals must result in thinking that is not governed by personal greeds and passions. Trying to see things "as they really are", that is in the context of the whole of reality, makes thinking bring everything into relation with the final goal of full knowledge or Enlightenment so that limited aims cease to dominate the mind's activity, which they do when the path is not followed. As a result of right thinking, wisdom gradually starts to develop. The whole life thus turns in the direction of the final goal and becomes a continuous training for its achievement.

3. *Right speech* (*sammā vāca*)

This and the next two parts of the path form practical guidelines for moralbehaviour in a man's personal and working life. They again follow naturally from the two previous steps, right viewing and right thinking, if these have been sufficiently deeply practised from the start. For newcomers to the path, however, explicit regulations and precepts were found to be unavoidable and they have to be followed scrupulously as long as one's understanding is undeveloped.

Right speech means abstaining from lying, from tale-bearing, from harsh language and from vain talk. Abstaining from lying is explained as never knowingly speaking a lie. Tale-bearing or repeating to others what one has heard somewhere else is almost always a cause for dissension and never serves a useful purpose from the spiritual point of view. Harsh language injures others and stems from an unkind or even malicious state of mind and has to be avoided. Vain talk means talking about irrelevant things, which is a waste of time and mental energy from the same point of view.

The positive formulation of right speech is: speaking only what is true; saying about others only what is praiseworthy; speaking only words that are gentle, soothing, loving, courteous and friendly; talking only about things that are useful, that lead to a better knowledge of reality, and promote morality and spiritual progress.

4. *Right acting* (*sammā kammanta*)

This is explained as abstention from killing, stealing, improper sexual conduct and taking intoxicants. As killing is always done for a purpose lower than the final goal of Enlightenment, ancient Buddhism does not admit any compromise for one who follows the path. Stealing or taking what has not been given must also be avoided, for again it can happen only when the mind is blinded by greed for things. Improper sexual conduct can be taken to be what is defined as such by the law and by the accepted moral values of a given society and is more strictly defined by special regulations for the community of monks (*Saṅgha*). Broadly speaking, a lay follower of the path avoids sex with those who are married to someone else, or are betrothed or under protection (of parents or the law), while monks abstain from sexual conduct altogether.

It should perhaps be pointed out here that the distinction between a lay follower and a monk (or nun) is rather a formal one. What really matters is the degree of the follower's inner commitment to the goal and the speed at which he wants to progress towards it. A Buddhist Yogi in modern times, especially if living in the West, may be fully committed to the path and a quick achievement of the goal, without necessarily giving it external expression by putting on monk's robes.

Intoxicants of all kinds are excluded because of their capacity to distort the processes of the mind, such as the ability to discriminate and to make sound judgments, and their tendency to cloud the clarity of perception and understanding and the possibility of developing higher vision through genuine meditation.

5. *Right livelihood* (*sammā ājīva*)

A follower of the Buddhist Yoga has to adopt a means of making his living which will not involve breaking the principles described above. In other words, he accepts his full personal responsibility for everything he does in the field of his professional activities. No order of a superior, no public demand, no loyalties of whatever kind can shift from the individual's shoulders the responsibility for offences against moral and spiritual principles (which are backed by the universal law of *karma*). This considerably narrows down the occupational options open to a strict follower of the path. The old texts mention some prohibited occupations such as those in which is involved, directly or indirectly, the destruction of life, telling untruths and any kind of trading where sex, arms, meat or intoxicants and poisons are involved. In complicated modern conditions careful individual thought and analysis have to be given to this subject, again according to the degree of the personal commitment.

6. *Right effort* (*sammā vāyāma*)

With this section of the path the actual Yoga training begins. The doctrinal formulation (usually called the "Four Great Efforts") calls for effort (1) to avoid unsuitable states of mind or (2) to overcome any that may have already entered the mind, (3) to develop suitable states of mind that one has not previously had and (4) to maintain those that one has already developed. Their suitability is measured by the way in which they are conducive to the final goal of Enlightenment.

The important message of this section of the Buddhist path is its clear indication of the importance and necessity of the element of will. Without the employment of volitional exertion there is no progress on the path of Yoga, no achievement of Enlightenment. Nor is it a matter of a decision to be made once and for all. The decision to carry on along the path has to be repeated and maintained from day to day and even from moment to moment. In other words, the volitional drive has to be steered in the direction of the goal until the vision of the goal becomes so clear and strong that deviation is virtually out of the question.

7. *Right mindfulness* (*sammā sati*)

This is the crucial section of the Buddhist eightfold path. Its objective is developing and training the mind in awareness. By introducing the element of constant watchful awareness of what is going on in the mind so that one is not a blind subject of mental forces or processes of which one knows very little or nothing, right mindfulness foreshadows Enlightenment itself, which is full knowledge of oneself as well as of reality as a whole.

The Yogi trains himself to keep his attention focused on his own actions, whether mental or bodily, in order to perform them in the full light of consciousness and not unaware, automatically or instinctually so that he might do something of which he would later disapprove. He tries to be constantly aware of what he is doing, feeling and thinking and of whatever other sorts of mental processes are going on in his mind. The result of this training is increasing self-knowledge and a growing capacity for acting according to his fully conscious will.

The actions and behaviour of nearly all people in everyday life seldom result from fully conscious decisions but are mostly determined by half conscious or unconscious reactions based on their character (which is composed of sets of habits, inclinations, instincts, urges and various other tendencies). These reactions are quite frequently in conflict with their own wishes when they have time to think about them and confront them with each other. This, however, happens extremely rarely, for with untrained individuals, reactions are usually followed quickly by actions prompted by them. Only when people suffer some grave and unpleasant consequences of their thoughtless actions do they become capable of considering the matter seriously and realise then, too late, that they in fact did not want to do what their reactions had driven them to.

On the other hand a Yogi trained in right mindfulness is able to see and distinguish the external stimuli, and the reactions to them which almost automatically arise in his mind, in the brief moment before the reactions can be translated into action. And this moment of clear insight into the working of his mind enables the trainee to preserve his control over it so that he can check those reactions and decide quite freely on action to be taken or on inaction, according to his knowledge or his long-held wishes or aspirations for higher aims. In the long run this procedure even enables him to change or completely drop certain habits or traits, to change and improve his whole character and finally to transcend the limitations of an individual personality altogether.

Buddhism has fully developed the methodical part of right mindfulness and also offers nowadays a number of techniques for meditational sessions as well as round-the-clock training in mindfulness. There is an abundant literature dealing with the subject, both old and modern.[1]

8. *Right absorption* (*sammā samādhi*)

The last section of the Buddhist path describes the progressive meditational achievements and experiences of a Yogi who dedicates his energies whole-heartedly to the cause of his spiritual development. The meditational procedure begins when the meditator withdraws his attention from the outer world and focuses it inside his mind. This process is achieved step by step while he is engaged in gradually dismissing and finally ignoring or even not noticing impressions entering his mind through the doors of the senses. Then he aims at freeing the mind from its preoccupation with ideas and images based on external data as well as from emotional involvements and conceptual problems. In the process of this gradual purging from the mind of material normally furnished to it by the senses, including the usually almost incessant flow of thinking based on sense information, and of ego-centred emotions and intellectual problems, the meditator eventually experiences a dynamic but burdenless state of mind often described as a pure and radiant stream of consciousness which has transcended both the external world of things and the internal world of the personal ego.

This gradual purification of the mind is described as proceeding through four stages of absorption (*jhānas*). The first one is still marked by an underlying process of mentation and sustained thought (*vittaka-vicāra*) which, however, is reduced to or concen-

1. The basic text for the study of the way of mindfulness (*sati*) is Satipaṭṭhāna Sutta (DN 22, MN 10), the commentary to it, and the relevant sections of Visuddhi Magga. Of modern expositions the following books are both well written and instructive :

Nyanaponika Thera : *The Heart of Buddhist Meditation*, London 1962.

E. H. Shattock : *An Experiment in Mindfulness*, London 1958.

Mahasi Sayadaw : *The Progress of Insight*, Kandy 1965.

,, ,, *Practical Insight Meditation*, Kandy 1971.

Sobhana Dhammasuddhi: *Insight Meditation*, 2nd ed., London 1968.

trated on one single object that has been chosen for the purpose of meditational training. When the mind is ready to relinquish this object and to leave behind even the last traces of thought process while still remaining alert and concentrated, the second stage of absorption is reached, in which the Yogi experiences a profound state of "enthusiasm", ecstasy or joy (*pīti*), stemming from the total unburdening of the mind, which has become emptied of all worldly concerns and thought activities. When, in the process of further meditations, the ecstasy of unburdening subsides, the third *jhāna* is entered into and the Yogi experiences only a subtle yet profound and intense feeling of happiness (*sukha*), which fills him entirely, but does not in the least disturb his calm. When this last experience has been enjoyed sufficiently and the Yogi is able to move beyond it, the fourth *jhāna* follows, which can be conceptually described only as complete equanimity (*upekkhā*), a "looking down" upon the teeming and eager life in *saṁsāra* without being attracted or perturbed by it. Yet even during this state of absorption the mind remains fully alert and watchful.

The fourth *jhāna* is the crucial achievement of the Buddhist Yoga. It is a state of alertness, equanimity and concentration which has to be understood as being beyond the grip of the normal saṁsāric world of duality, while not being completely outside it. One can describe it figuratively as being only a step away from the final goal of *Nirvāṇa*, although it is not actually linked to *Nirvāṇa* and need not necessarily be followed by it. The fourth absorption is like a threshold between *saṁsāra* and *Nirvāṇa*. From it the world of *saṁsāra* can be contemplated and scrutinised as a whole as well as in its details, and from it the final breakthrough to Enlightenment can also be accomplished.

But in order to crown the Buddhist eightfold path with the highest achievement of true knowledge or wisdom and true liberation, which is what, in effect, Enlightenment represents to us as far as we can appreciate its meaning, all the parts of the path will have to have been brought to perfection: those dealing with morality (3, 4, 5), those concerned with the meditational evolution of the mind (6, 7, 8), and those that constitute wisdom (1, 2)—wisdom, however, that is based on an accomplished metaphysical vision and realisation, meaning wisdom or complete knowledge that is not a possession, but the unity of knowing and being.

This accomplishment can be reached only when the meditational absorptions have been supplemented by the progress of insight (*vipassanā*) brought to perfection. There are therefore two basic lines running through the Buddhist Yoga training : the development of tranquillity in the mind (called technically *samatha bhāvanā*) through the four stages of absorption as described by the eighth part of the path, and the development of insight (*vipassanā bhāvanā*) as methodically elaborated by the seventh part of the path.

It is, then, the combination of the two lines of training—which may take variegated forms with innumerable variations—that eventually brings about the perfect achievement. Right absorption (*samādhi*) alone, even when brought to perfection, cannot in itself bring the final result of liberation. The development of insight or the perfection of mindfulness (*sati*), on the other hand, requires only a certain approximation to full absorption (called by Pāli commentators *upacāra samādhi*) before the final wisdom and liberation are reached. The four *jhānas* need not be fully developed.[1]

## 2. THE YOGA OF PATAÑJALI

The Yoga system handed down under the name of Patañjali and presented in the slender volume of his Yoga Sūtras (which,

1. A systematic description of the Buddhist methods of meditation is given in the following book :

Vajiraññāṇa Mahāthera : *Buddhist Meditation in Theory and Practice*, Colombo 1962.

It seems that the modern Buddhist schools of meditation favour the path of insight (*vipassanā bhāvanā*) without cultivating full absorptions. On the other hand, most reports of the Pāli Canon about the Buddha's disciples who achieved *Nirvāṇa* show that the combination of full *samatha bhāvanā* and *vipassanā bhāvanā* was preferred. But no disciple seems to have fully repeated the Buddha's achievement of Enlightenment with the full vision of totality (the whole saṁsāric cycle of life etc.). a feat which later became the *piè ce de résistance* of the Mahāyānists.

The experience of *samādhi* as the result of *samatha bhāvanā* training is more complex than described in this chapter. Apart from the four concrete absorptions (*rūpa jhānas*) described here, there are also four abstract absorptions (*arūpa jhānas*) and the achievement of suspension (*nirodha samāpatti*). To simplify the matter for this survey I have not discussed these as they are not vital to the early Buddhist Yoga.

however, is practically always edited together with bulky commentaries) has gained the reputation of being *the* classical exposition of Yoga. It is sometimes referred to as Rāja Yoga, which can be translated as the "royal path".

Patañjali's Yoga is the second of the systematic or integral expositions of the Yoga technique that have been preserved from ancient times. It is possible to say that upon the whole it is more elaborate and summarises the actual technique of Yoga procedures more exactly than the Buddhist exposition. This is probably due to the fact that Patañjali's Yoga Sūtras are of the nature of a technical manual, whereas the Buddhist exposition is incorporated in live discourses of the Buddha with his disciples.

As to the time and the personality of the author of the Yoga Sūtras, full agreement has not yet been reached among scholars because of the lack of decisive evidence and the scarcity of reliable material on which to base definite views. Virtually nothing is known about Patañjali himself, and not even legendary data have been handed down. In this respect the difference between him and the creator of the first integral Yoga system, the Buddha, cannot be greater. There are other obvious differences, too. The Buddha was the founder of his system, even though, admittedly, he made use of some of the experiences he had previously gained under various Yoga teachers of the time. Patañjali was neither a founder nor a leader of a new movement or community and his personality in no way emerges from his text, which is very short, condensed and impersonal. On analysis we see that he put nothing into it that had not been known before and he did not aim at creating anything new. The ingenuity of his achievement lies in the thoroughness and completeness with which all the important stages of Yoga practice and mental experiences are included in his scheme, and in their systematic presentation in a succinct treatise. Patañjali was a codifier of what was best in the Yoga practice and knowledge of his time.

His time cannot, however, be determined with any degree of accuracy. He was certainly post-Buddhist, although views have been expressed to the contrary,[1] and it is hardly possible to place him much before the starting-point of our era, although some place him several centuries later.[2] From various discussions of the problem the resulting impression is that the composition of Patañjali's Yoga Sūtras could have taken place any time between 300 B.C. and 300 A.D. What is beyond doubt, however, is that the material the Sūtras contain dates back before this period and some of it even before the time of the Buddha. There are probably also one or two later interpolations in the text of the Sūtras, particularly in its polemical part, which can be dated to the fourth or fifth century A.D.[3] Some authors also have made it seem most likely that the text of the Sūtras is not a unitary work, but combines into one whole two or even three originally separate texts.[4] This again only confirms that the final redactor of the text, whoever he was, was not and did not intend to be an original author of a new teaching, but simply created a systematic presentation of the Yoga lore of his time.

The methodical scheme of Patañjali's Yoga has—like that of the Buddha—eight parts. All of them had been known before Patañjali and their gradual emergence and even the process of ordering them into a sequence almost identical with that of the Yoga Sūtras can be followed in the Yoga Upaniṣads.

The Yoga Upaniṣads do not belong to the group of the oldest Brāhmanical Upaniṣadic texts in which mythology, symbology and philosophical speculation are combined with a kind of metaphysical vision, sometimes based on meditational absorption (*dhyāna*—see Chānd. Up. VII, 6, 1), but their contents are based on an equally old tradition, which developed in the

1. Cf. Hariharānanda Āraṇya : *Yoga Philosophy of Patañjali*, Calcutta 1963, p. 4.

2. J. H. Woods concludes that the Sūtras must have been written between 300 and 500 A.D. See his *The Yoga System of Patañjali*, Harvard Uni. Press, repr. Delhi 1966, pp. xvii-xix.

3. For a summarised discussion of the problem of dating the Yoga Sūtras, see Eliade, *Yoga, Immortality and Freedom*, pp. 370-372.

4. This view had already been expressed by Deussen, *Allg. Gesch. d. Phil.* I, 3, pp. 507 ff. and is further discussed and supported by J.W. Hauer, *Yoga. Ein indischer Weg zum Selbst*, pp. 223 ff.

main outside the brāhmanical circles in the communities and schools of non-orthodox ascetics. As the Brāhmanical quest for the experience of the Ultimate grew important, at least in some quarters, and found acceptance among spiritually-minded Brāhmans as being higher than the practice of traditional sacrifices, the independent Yoga tradition penetrated more and more into the Upaniṣads, the Śvetāśvatara and Kaṭha being the best illustrations of this trend. There are even sections of these Upaniṣads already describing the Yoga path or practice, which gradually acquires a systematic form. For instance, Kaṭha Upaniṣad mentions the basic requirements of Yoga practice, such as the withdrawal of the mind's attention from the senses (*pratyāhāra*) and the training in the concentration of the mind (*dhāraṇā*) with the subsequent unification of the mind with the ultimate reality (*samādhi*). Even different stages of samādhi are described.[1] Śvetāśvatara Upaniṣad is even more explicit in its description of the Yoga path, although it is not presented systematically there. But it even mentions physical constituents of the Yoga practice: *āsana* (position) and *prāṇāyāma* (regulation of breathing), in addition to the mental ones: *pratyāhāra, dhāraṇā, dhyāna* and *samādhi*. Those subsequent Upaniṣads that specialise in Yoga and are therefore known as Yoga Upaniṣads elaborate on various aspects of Yoga practice and deal also with philosophical and religious elements that often accompany Yoga practice, according to the school to which each particular Upaniṣad belongs.

The Yoga Sūtras of Patañjali appeared during a time when Yoga was no longer the practice of a few, but had become very popular as a result of the spread of Buddhism, Jainism, and other unorthodox schools and of the acceptance of Yoga on the part of orthodox religious circles who modified Yoga practice and interpretation to suit their respective sectarian cults and beliefs. This led inevitably to the loosening of some strict Yoga rules and principles of practice. In particular the principle of the purification of the mind as a preparation for a higher spiritual vision was too much influenced by sectarian ideas and imagery and the goal became the achievement of

7. See Kaṭha Up., especially chap. 3 and 6.

ecstatic union with one's chosen deity (*iṣṭa devatā*). This in turn led in some cases to a less strict observance cf the moral discipline current in ascetic and Yoga schools, and in extreme cases even led to its obliteration. In this situation Patañjali's text set standards for the practice and aims of Yoga which—while allowing some space for different conceptions of the nature of existence, the final goal and the role, if any, of God in Yoga—were so impressive and found such strong consensus that they could not easily be disregarded. The Yoga Sūtras therefore came to be viewed as a classical text of Yoga and have remained so practically till the present day. They represent the strict, sober and sincere trend in Yoga as it was followed by generations of earnest truth-seekers over many centuries, a trend that had previously found expression only in the Buddha's eightfold path, from which Patañjali obviously benefited. His eightfold path (*aṣṭānga yoga*) can be summarised as follows :

1. *Yama.* This word may be interpreted as "abstinence". It represents the conscious endeavour on the part of the Yogi to abstain from doing things that keep his mind involved in the indiscriminate struggle for survival and satisfaction within the existing scale of values in life. Although the stress seems to lie on abstaining, which is a negative concept, the contents of the "abstinences" are sometimes positive. They are five in number:

(1) *Ahiṁsā* means non-violence, abstaining from killing and hurting other beings.

(2) *Satya* is truthfulness and implies abstaining from telling lies and from falseness of any kind.

(3) *Asteya* means abstaining from stealing.

(4) *Brahmacarya*, literally "divine faring", means living in accordance with the standards of the goal of Yoga, which is union with God or with the ultimate reality, or the final direct knowledge thereof (depending on interpretation). Therefore those associations that impede progress towards the goal owing to the overwhelming impact they may have on the mind and the whole personality have to be renounced. Sexual union has been regarded as the most powerful diverting influence of this kind and has therefore been avoided by serious fully-

committed Yogis. *Brahmacarya* therefore became synonymous with chastity or celibacy.

(5) *Aparigraha* may be interpreted as "abstaining from appropriating". It is an attitude of mind that does not consider anything to be one's own, even if one is using it (such as the physical body) and even if it seems to be essential for life (including "one's own" life).

(2) *Niyama.* Both *yama* and *niyama* are words derived from the same root "yam" which, as a verb, means to control, to tame. *Niyama* can be interpreted as "observance" and it represents the Yogi's progressive effort to observe certain principles that prepare his personality for achievements of a higher order. They are also five in number :

(1) *Śauca* means purity and it is external as well as internal. The Yogi has to strive for pure thinking, speaking and acting, to keep his body clean, see to the purity of his food, act from pure motives and cleanse his mind of sensuality and urges.

(2) *Santoṣa* is contentment. It expresses the willingness of the Yogi to accept and face reality as it is without being elated or depressed by it. He has to bear equally pleasure and pain, gain and loss, fame and contempt, success and failure, sympathy and hostility. He must be able, if necessary, to reduce his needs to the bare necessities of life.

(3) *Tapas* means traditionally "austerity" and introduces into the practice of Yoga forbearance, fasts and other ascetic practices that help to reduce the Yogi's dependence on things that cannot be altogether avoided, but should not become desirable for their own sake. In this way he increases his self-control.

(4) *Svādhyāya* is self-development or self education and points to the necessity of continuous study, constant learning and development of one's intelligence and higher mental faculties.

(5) *Īśvarapraṇidhāna* may be interpreted as "constant thought of the Divine" (a more literal rendering is "surrender to the Lord"). It is an admonition to be constantly aware that there is the transcendent, which the Yogi may not yet have experienced, but which is his goal and which

should therefore be constantly in his mind, accompanying all his thoughts and actions.

3. *Āsana* means "position", "posture". For efficient Yoga practice it is essential to be able to assume a stable and agreeable position when training the mind so that the mind is free from bodily interference, which normally compels one to move or change position. In India since time immemorial it has been a cross-legged position. It has several varieties of which the lotus posture (*padmāsana*) is the most impressive one.

4. *Prāṇāyāma* is the control of the process of breathing. It is usually done in the position chosen for Yoga practice. It regulates breathing and its rhythm, especially by slowing it down and also by introducing longer breaks between the phases of breathing. Since there is a close connection between the flow of respiration and the dynamics of the mind, the help which can thereby be obtained in establishing some balance of mind, enhancing its clarity and capacity for observation, is considerable.

5. *Pratyāhāra* means "withdrawal". It is the first purely mental step in this system of Yoga, aiming as it does at preparing the mind for spiritual vision, which can come from within only when the mind becomes receptive in that direction rather than expecting everything to enter it from outside in a similar way to all the information about the external world. A mind made clear and calm by *prāṇāyāma* is now further purified by withdrawing its attention from the activity of the senses, which normally constantly fill it with images derived from external objects. The withdrawal of attention from the senses cuts off the flow of perceptions created by external objects and the mind can then be trained in the succeeding steps of the path, which involve the technique of opening it to inner vision.

6. *Dhāraṇā* means concentration and its aim is to bring about "one-pointedness" (*ekāgratā*) of the mind, which can then stay focused on one particular object of its (internal) experience in a way unknown to the mind when it operates on the level of sense data. This concentration also results in a degree of understanding and comprehension of the chosen object that eventually penetrates into its very essence or nature.

7. *Dhyāna* may be translated as contemplation or absorption. It is reached when concentration becomes spontaneous. It is then a natural process for the mind of the Yogi, just as thinking is natural for everybody else, so that no special effort is needed to embark on it. At this stage the penetration of the essence of the object of contemplation becomes complete. This technique then enables the mind to approach reality as such "from inside" which is the suprasensory and supraintellectual, direct way of cognition. This leads to the final achievement.

8. *Samādhi*, which may be translated as unification. Samādhi is the crown of Yoga endeavours in Patañjali's system. It is the fully conscious and "factual" unification of the Yogi's vision or cognitive capacity or mind itself with the heart of reality in its wholeness which sets him free. He reaches final liberation from the bondage to limited forms of existence that can exist only through ignorance or lack of total vision. But *samādhi* is not a simple experience. It is realised in stages. The sequence and relationship of these stages is not entirely clear from Patañjali's text. It is also quite possible that in practice the stages cannot be fully distinguished from one another and that they are simply a broad guide for the Yogi to measure his progress approximately before he reaches the final goal. However, some tentative picture of the stages of progress through *samādhi* has to be given.

Firstly, there appears to be a broad division of the experience of samādhi into two categories : (1) unification still based on the process of conceiving (*samprajñāta samādhi*) and (2) unification beyond the process of conceiving (*asamprajñāta samādhi*). Unification based on conceiving has itself several stages. To start with, there is the "inside" unification with the object of meditation (which, of course, is no longer felt to be an object in the ordinary sense), accompanied by the process of understanding its dynamic nature. This stage might be called (i) "intelligible unification" (*savitarka samādhi*). This then changes into a state in which the object is in the full light of knowledge; it is known simultaneously in all its aspects and inner dimensions so that although it appears to us that the act of knowing must imply an experience of duration, here it does not seem to be a process in time. Perhaps we can interpret this second stage as (ii) "unification beyond intelligibility" (*nirvitarka samādhi*). Henceforth grasp of the object seems to move from the level of individual things into the realm of what we may call archetypes (borrowing C.G. Jung's expression). The object is grasped in its archetypal (tanmātric) setting. Perhaps this stage may be called (iii) "ideational unification" (*savicāra samādhi*). Further understanding of what the object really is in the context of the ultimate reality that is beyond archetypes or ideas (in Plato's sense) might be called (iv) "unification beyond ideation" (*nirvicāra samādhi*).

The stages of unification are accompanied by experiences on a high emotional level. They become particularly noticeable during *nirvicāra samādhi* and are of the nature of bliss (*ānanda*). This bliss has to be regarded as a very subtle and highly spiritual experience. Perhaps we can look upon it as a parallel phenomenon to the experience of joy on the ordinary level when living in the cognitive domain of the senses and intellect where emotional experiences of joy and elation often accompany creative intellectual activity, particularly accomplished cognitive achievements, such as the creation of a new scientific theory. The suprasensory and supraintellectual universe need not, and perhaps must not, be viewed as emotionally colourless. Spiritual bliss of some kind is an accompanying factor in practically all known forms of mysticism as well as in Yoga and Buddhism. It obviously compensates for the renunciation of the basic pleasures and joys of life on an everyday level, a compensation that seems to be more than adequate.

When the Yogi's mind is, as described, elated, purified and unified in the process of directly knowing the innermost nature of the object in its fullness and in the (tanmātric) context of the whole of reality "from within", he becomes aware also of his own status, his "selfhood" (*asmitā*). In other words, he penetrates to the centre or essence of himself as he did in the case of the whole of reality.

As an analysis of everyday experience shows, the I-consciousness is evasive and without a permanent seat, constantly shifting according to the kind of experience that prevails at any given moment. The result is that when speaking about himself, man identifies himself sometimes with his body (e.g. "I am tall"), sometimes with his emotions ("I am angry") and at other times with various mental processes (e.g. "I think"). Now, in the stage of absorption described, the Yogi is supposed to find the evasive centre of his I-consciousness, the dimension of his self-hood.[1]

The Yogi who has gone through all the previous stages, starting with the withdrawal of his attention from his senses (*pratyāhāra*) continuing by applying his concentration (*dhāraṇā*) to a chosen meditational object and then deepening his experience into a state of inner contemplation (*dhyāna*), has now in the complex experience of *samādhi* reached the last station of his journey in this world. He has penetrated to the essence of his own being and he also has come to the point of knowing reality in its wholeness—not confronting it as a vast object, but knowing it by a cognitive-cum-existential process of inner unification. That is why *samādhi* has to be understood as having an epistemological as well as an ontological character, as being a "unification in cognition" or "cognition by unification". This is what is probably expressed by the qualifying attribute *samprajñāta* which we rendered as "based on the process of conceiving", however subtle and difficult to imagine such conceiving may be in the state of *nirvicāra samādhi*.

When the full impact of this "last station" is realised, it gives the Yogi the power of all-knowledge (*sarvajñatṛtva*)—quite logically, for it is his pure self's experience of universality. In its perfect form this highest experience is called *dharma-megha-samādhi* which might be interpreted or circumscribed as "epistemological-cum-ontological unification" (*samādhi*) with the wholeness (*megha*) of reality (*dharma*). This must be the full, direct and final global vision of truth and it represents a point of saturation from which there is nowhere else or nowhere further to go. But at the same time this state appears to be of a highly unstable character and it cannot last, it does not represent some sort of "realm of metaphysical Being". This fullness cannot be kept nor is there any reason for wanting to keep it. So the next step following this point of saturation, the only possible and logical

1. Commentaries to Patañjali's Sūtras, particularly that of Vyāsa, regard the bliss experience and pure self (or pure I) experience as two distinct stages of absorption (as *ānanda samādhi* and *asmitā samādhi* respectively).

outcome of the situation is the abandonment or transcending of the last trace of what may still be viewed as mental process, albeit its contents are the heart and fullness of reality.

What follows then is still *samādhi*, but without any trace of conceiving (*asamprajñāta samādhi*), which is beyond comprehension. It frees the Yogi's mind from the last remnant of contents anchored in the process of experiencing. In this absolute absence of anything conceivable, the real status of the self (*puruṣa*) is discovered and the result is total freedom or deliverance (*mokṣa*); final and complete autonomy or "isolation" (*kaivalya*) from categories of existence is won.

The Yogi who has realised this total freedom of the self during his lifetime is looked upon as a "living saint" (*jīvanmukta*).[1]

### 3. FURTHER SCHOOLS OF YOGA

The two systems of integral Yoga practice, that of the Buddha and that of Patañjali, are the culminations of Yoga endeavours, trends and traditions stretching from the remote past and pursued for centuries outside the official stream of the Brāhmanic culture. But when they reached their peaks, they became very conspicuous and, consequently, visible to all, including ordinary people whose religious loyalty became diverted from Brāhmans to Yogis and wandering ascetics. As a result, in the subsequent movement of Brāhmanic revivalism, some of the Yogic methodical principles and guidelines to spiritual life as well as the aim of Yoga—direct experience of the ultimate reality—became

1. There are many books and treatises dealing with Patañjali's Yoga (quite often together with Sāṅkhya philosophy), but a scholarly work which would give a thorough analysis and balanced interpretation is still missing. The following is a selection of important works for study :

R. Garbe : *Samkhya und Yoga*, Strassburg 1898.

S. Dasgupta : *A Study of Patañjali*, Calcutta 1920.

,, *Yoga as Philosophy and Religion*, London 1924.

,, *Yoga Philosophy in Relation to Other Systems of Indian Thought*. Calcutta 1930.

J.H. Woods : *The Yoga System of Patañjali*, repr. Delhi 1966.

Hariharananda Āranya : *Yoga Philosophy of Patañjali*, Calcutta 1963.

G. Coster : *Yoga and Western Psychology*, London 1934, repr. Delhi 1968.

I.K. Taimni : *The Science of Yoga*, Adyar 1965.

generally accepted as the higher strata of religious life open to anybody who wanted to tread such a path. Thus Yoga became an inseparable part of Brāhmanism or Hinduism and the great swing towards its popularisation began. Naturally, the religious element made itself strongly felt in this development so that some Yogic movements acquired a trait which in other religious traditions is invariably called mysticism.[1]

The best codification of the popularised Yoga path at the end of which lies union with God is the Bhagavad Gītā. Although a popularisation, the presentation of Yoga and its various aspects and methods in the Bhagavad Gītā has a certain depth that makes it the most recognised and cherished text for most Indian God-seekers and its fame has become, in modern times, world-wide. The Bhagavad Gītā has implanted the seed of Yoga, over many centuries, in the minds and hearts of vast multitudes that otherwise would not have been touched by it. These multitudes no doubt grasped the message of Yoga only partially. However, this grasp created a unique situation in India and engendered an atmosphere of spiritual quest in which recurrent peaks of achievement have been possible.

The appeal of the Yoga of the Bhagavad Gītā is perhaps due to the way in which it is presented, with various aspects of Yoga being treated almost as separate types of Yoga. These subsequently developed their respective methodological features still further and practically constituted themselves into separate schools of Yoga. The most important ones are four in number: Karma Yoga, Dhyāna Yoga, Jñāna Yoga and Bhakti Yoga.

*Karma Yoga* is the path of action. The Bhagavad Gītā discusses it mainly in the third chapter and its justification seems to be based there on two main ideas. Firstly it is suggested that even when one enters on the spiritual path it is not possible to abstain altogether from active participation in life, and secondly it is argued that action arises, in fact, from *Brahman*, the source of all manifested

1. It goes without saying that this trend had its prehistory. A religious Yoga tradition focused on the idea of God (Brahma) as the highest reality must have existed before. Although the Buddha either ignored it or put it into perspective as not leading to the ultimate (*Nirvāṇa* according to Buddhism is far beyond Brahmic dimensions), Patañjali respected it as is shown by the sections of the Sūtras which deal with Īśvara.

being. Thus action is something which man shares with the Divine. The problems lie in what sort of action one should perform, what its motivation should be and how it should be performed. An action motivated by selfish desire (*kāma*) or anger (*krodha*) leads to evil and blinds man so that he cannot see wisdom and can only act foolishly.

The remedy that Karma Yoga offers lies in the renunciation of personal aims when acting. To live for satisfaction based on sensual pleasure and external achievements is to live in vain. Such a life is entirely wasted. One should and can find pleasure, satisfaction and contentment in oneself (for there is the universal *Ātman* to be found eventually) and then there is nothing one has to do exclusively for one's own interest. Works, whether done or undone, do not then touch one who is not dependent on their results. Such a person does, without attachment, whatever is correct under the circumstances. His actions are directed by concern for the welfare and coherence of the world.

In this way he becomes like the Divine, that issues the world and sustains it, although there is no need for the Divine to do so and no motivation can be ascribed to the Divine. When a man acts like this, his works do not bind him and he will find release from the world of action.

*Dhyāna Yoga* is the path of meditation. Firstly it is made clear that the spiritual path of meditation does not necessarily lead to withdrawal from engagement in actions in the world. The quietude which the Yogi usually seeks in renouncing life in the world is, in fact, won more safely by renouncing the aim (*saṅkalpa*) of life in the world, while remaining active in it. For what really counts is the mental attitude. One can renounce the world and involvement in its affairs externally and yet remain bound by worldly ties in one's mind, if only negatively by fighting and suppressing the memories or fresh opportunities of worldly involvement. But if one succeeds, in one's mind, in giving up personal benefit or expectations thereof as motivation for one's actions, no involvement in active life in the world will disturb one's inner balance needed for successful meditation. In other words, Dhyāna Yoga or the path of meditation can be pursued while man is engaged in a worldly life, provided he also practises

Karma Yoga or the path of renunciation of the personal fruits of actions. In this way the lower self of man becomes ruled by his higher self and his personality becomes harmonised and integrated. His meditational efforts will then be crowned with success.

The Bhagavad Gītā even gives methodical advice for the Dhyāna practice of Yoga while remaining in the world. For the purpose of meditation a person has to retire regularly for a given period of time into a quiet place, be seated comfortably and withdraw attention from his environment by directing the gaze of his eyes to his nose-tip. Breathing is kept regular and smooth and the thinking process of the mind is checked so that eventually "one-pointedness" is achieved. In this state the Yogi then approaches *Brahman* and in the end experiences the peace which the Bhagavad Gītā calls, like the early Buddhist texts did, *Nirvāṇa* and which is, according to it, rooted in the Divine.

*Jñāna Yoga* is the path of knowledge. In the last instance this knowledge becomes wisdom or the final direct realisation of the essential unity of existence. At the same time, however, the eternal existence of the person (*puruṣa*) of the Yogi is maintained even in liberation. This is a mystery that Jñāna Yoga proposes to solve by direct experience, not by knowing the solution conceptually. That is why the Bhagavad Gītā does not really claim to expound this final knowledge, but only advises that everything should be seen as stemming from the Divine, which is therefore to be sought as the changeless essence behind changing forms.

The view of the essential oneness behind phenomena, expressed fully and openly in the Upaniṣads and made popular by the Bhagavad Gītā, was later philosophically elaborated by Śankara in his Advaita Vedānta system of thought. He also gave practical instructions concerning Yoga techniques so that a summary of Jñāna Yoga methodology can be attempted on the basis of Śankara's writings[1] where the Bhagavad Gītā leaves us without systematic guidance. Śankara was not only a philo-

1. Mainly from his *Brahmasūtrabhāṣya*. A short summary is given by E. Deutsch in his *Advaita Vedānta*, pp. 105-6.

sopher, but also, among other things, a practising Yogi and a founder of a distinct monastic tradition of Advaita Yogis.

There are four basic requirements in the Jñāna Yoga discipline in which the Yogi has to train himself:

1. *Viveka* (discrimination). The aspirant has to develop and cultivate the ability to recognise what is impermanent, temporary and fleeting in life as he experiences it, and what is of lasting value and pointing to the eternal. He has to try to discriminate between the superficial and the essential, between the illusory reality on the surface and the absolute reality in the inner, deep dimension of existence. In this way he has to try to scrutinise, analyse and evaluate constantly his experiences, inclinations, decisions and actions.

2. *Vairāgya* (dispassionateness). The Yogi has to guard his mind against becoming possessed, infatuated or, later, even slightly disturbed by passions springing from sensual desires; or from attachment to things that bring sensual satisfaction. *Rāga* means originally "colouring", which indicates that passions are, in fact, obstructions of the mind that do not allow clear vision. To achieve the clarity of mind that is essential for final knowledge and wisdom, attachments and passions that "colour" it so that it sees distortedly must be got rid of.

3. *Ṣaṭsampatti* (six attainments). This instruction contains a programme of self-education for success on the Yoga path covering six points:

(1) *Śama* or the cultivation of tranquillity of the mind.

(2) *Dama* or self-control in acting.

(3) *Uparati* or eradicating the eagerness to possess.

(4) *Titikṣā* or patience.

(5) *Śraddhā* or confidence, also meaning sincerity.

(6) *Samādhāna* or intentness of the mind.

4. *Mumukṣatva* ("longing for liberation"). This last requirement is very important. The aspirant must develop a positive longing (not to say a passion) for liberation. Its development is supported by the previous endeavours as described above, especially by the advanced ability to discriminate between the unsatisfactory superficial reality and the safety-promising, spiritual dimension of higher experience.

The training of the Jñāna Yogi of the Advaita Vedānta tradition proceeds, generally speaking, through three stages:
1. *Śravaṇa.* This means "hearing". The aspirant has first to go through a period of extensive and intensive study, which in ancient times was done by listening to the teachings of his master. Nowadays it includes thorough studies of the traditional doctrines of the Upaniṣads and the Advaitic texts, particularly Śankara's commentaries, either "at the feet of a master" or by reading. This should give the mind of the aspirant the right direction and outlook and material for the next stage:
2. *Manana.* This can be translated as thinking or "mentation". It starts with intellectual analysis of the material gained by studying the texts. The analysis is then applied to the aspirant's knowledge of the world and himself and this enables him to realize that within the world of sensual and emotional experience and on the level of speculative thinking final knowledge cannot be found. Absolute truth can lie only beyond them. When he firmly arrives at this conclusion, he is able to enter the path of meditation which brings him to the following and final stage of training:
3. *Nididhyāsana.* This expression can be translated as "constant meditation". This stage of training makes it clear to the aspirant that the process of opening a new channel to reality over and above the senses and the intellect is not a matter of mental exercises during meditational sessions only, but that it is also and equally necessary to introduce a kind of meditational attitude into one's life so that eventually the mind is in a state of meditation even when dealing with the business of everyday living. As this capacity is developed and deepened, the Yogi's intuition and spiritual vision grow until he reaches the final vision of truth, which brings him the final achievement of liberation (*mokṣa*).

*Bhakti Yoga* or the path of Divine love is perhaps the only Yoga school based entirely on belief in a personal God as the highest goal of man's spiritual pilgrimage. It is true that some other schools of Yoga also accept the existence of God (often called *Īśvara*—the Lord), but they do not ascribe to him the mark of ultimateness. Thus even Buddhism accepts the existence of a Brahma as the highest being within this universe, who lives in luminous spiritual spheres and possesses a very noble mind and immense power. He can survey the universe with its diverse spheres of life and can be of assistance to beings lower in status than himself, including those who are struggling along their spiritual paths. Among Buddhist meditational devices for the development of the four concrete absorptions (*rūpa jhānas*) there is one called the "Four Divine Abodes" (*Brahma vihāras*) in which the objects meditated on are the qualities ascribed to the divine character of a Brahma. They are love (*mettā*), compassion (*karuṇā*), sympathetic joy (*muditā*) and equanimity (*upekkhā*).

But these achievements, although very high, do not, in themselves, represent one single step towards final liberation or liberating knowledge, if not supplemented by special "insight" meditation. They are, of course, the best possible preparation for the development of wisdom: the fourth absorption, characterised by complete tranquillity of mind, is the best basis for insight meditation (*vipassanā bhāvanā*). But here the assistance, help or encouragement that a thought of Brahma may provide ends, for he himself is viewed in Buddhism as being ignorant of the higher path of insight and the spiritual achievements and spheres it leads to. He himself has to follow the Buddha's eightfold path, otherwise in due course he will inevitably lose his high position as a result of samsāric changes and be reborn sooner or later in a lower sphere of life.

In Patañjali's Yoga system also the Lord (*Īśvara*) plays only a limited part, although his status is understood to be higher there than in the Buddhist system. The whole outline of the eightfold Yoga path shows that it was designed without reliance on a higher personality, such as God, as a helper. It is based on recognition of the existence of a reliable spiritual law (no doubt inherited from the Vedic notion of *ṛta*). However, in accordance with the religious beliefs and traditions of the time, the Lord was recognised even within Patañjali's system as being of considerable help to those who had faith in him and were therefore inspired by thinking of him on their Yoga path. His status is described in the Sūtras, in accordance with the teachings of Sāṅkhya philosophy, as one of eternal freedom. He is not, however, the creator or cause of the existence of the universe or other beings. He is just one of the innumerable number of eternal personalities (*puruṣas*) like any other being in the universe, only, unlike all other beings, he has never been entangled in saṁsāric (phenomenal) existence. When a Yogi is inspired by the idea of the existence of an eternally pure being, the *Īśvara*, without actually doing anything himself, in a way helps the Yogi out of *saṁsāra*. This could be called a kind of *Bhakti* relationship. We can understand that love for a person can inspire achievements in man without the loved person's doing anything directly to assist. However, the Yogi has to go through all the stages of the Yoga training like anyone else.

In the Bhagavad Gītā the notion of a personal God as the highest reality is underlined by the doctrine of Divine incarnations (*avatāras*). Kṛṣṇa appears there to be one of them, while being fully aware also of his eternal nature. He does recognise the Yoga paths that lead directly to the transcendental, imperishable and unmanifest ultimate reality, but says that they are too difficult and only for a few, and that even they lead, in fact, to him. It seems that what is being hinted at here without any attempt to discuss the question philosophically is the mystery of the nature of the ultimate which, while it is often spoken of as being impersonal or beyond all concepts of personality as understood by the human mind, yet at the same time possesses all that we associate with the notion of a supreme personality called God or the Lord. As such it can be approached not only by the few philosophically-minded practising Yogis, but also by multitudes.

The path towards the ultimate viewed as the Lord then becomes a life of devotional surrender of the worshipper to a particular manifested form of the divine Lord. Every thought, emotion, word and deed becomes an act of sacrifice directed towards him. This unrestrained devotion should in the end bring a liberation as definite as the methodical Yoga paths of other types. The practice of the Yoga of devotion or Bhakti Yoga is variegated and it is hardly possible to describe it in a systematic way or find in it a well-defined methodical approach. In this respect Bhakti Yoga resembles Christian mysticism or Islamic sufism more than the classical schools of Indian Yoga.

To make this chapter more complete a few other types of Yogic techniques must be mentioned which are not, in themselves, separate schools of Yoga, but elaborations of some aspects or stages as they occur in the course of integral Yoga practice. Of these techniques Haṭha Yoga has become nowadays the most popular.

*Haṭha Yoga* may be viewed as a further elaborate extension of the third and fourth parts of Patañjali's Yoga system, namely that concerned with the bodily posture (*āsana*) and that dealing with the control of breathing (*prāṇāyāma*). Nothing is known about any elaborate system of bodily positions in Patañjali's time apart from several variations of the cross-legged sitting posture, and little is known about the techniques of the breathing exercises, although they undoubtedly existed in Patañjali's time and even earlier. But the beginning of the whole system of Haṭha Yoga is still obscure.[1] Nowadays it comprises three main disciplines; a sequence of intricate bodily positions, a number of procedures for the purification of the body internally, and numerous complicated breathing exercises.

All sources seem to agree that Haṭha Yoga is a useful if not entirely necessary introduction to higher Yoga of some kind and that it cannot lead to the realization of higher truth on its own. But it is maintained that it greatly increases the chance of subsequent spiritual progress when a mental Yoga path is taken up. The system of bodily positions is supposed to have been designed in order to bring about perfect physiological harmony in the organism, which amounts to perfect health and efficiency. In the process of bodily training the mind is trained as well, for the Yogi develops through it a high degree of self-control and determination and learns the technique of self-observation, which leads to the heightening of the capacity of awareness. Great emphasis is laid also on the influence of the exercises on the nervous system whose sensitivity is further enhanced by the purificatory procedures.

1. The three oldest known Sanskrit texts that are the sources for *Haṭha Yoga* (*Gheraṇḍa Saṃhitā*, *Śiva Saṃhitā* and *Haṭha Yoga Pradīpikā*) date from mediaeval times. But there are indications that they are based on older sources at present unknown to us. There is also evidence showing that breathing exercises were practised in the Buddha's time and earlier.

One of the best modern books about *Haṭha Yoga* is : Theos Bernard : *Haṭha Yoga*, London 1950.

The protracted practice of complicated breathing exercises is meant to influence the working of the mind towards increasing its ability to concentrate, and some of them are designed to produce ecstatic states of mind or trances. It is further believed that the breathing exercises activate the subtle vital energy of the body which is in fact the cosmic life-force (*prāṇa*) which sustains man and through which he is linked to the universal or cosmic dimension of life.

*Kuṇḍalinī Yoga.* An occult superstructure to which Haṭha Yoga may lead those who feel inclined to go that way is called Kuṇḍalinī Yoga. Its basis is an elaborate and complicated teaching that describes in great detail the physiology of man's subtle body, which is supposed to be the vehicle of the cosmic life-force (*prāṇa*). The teaching on one or more subtle and mental bodies or "sheaths" of man (*śarīras, kāyas or kośas*) apart from the physical one is very old and mentioned clearly in some Upaniṣads and also in the Buddhist Pāli Canon.

The theory goes that certain Haṭha Yoga positions practised in a particular way and combined with further exercises called *mudrās* awaken the dormant spiritual energy called *Kuṇḍalinī* which normally rests coiled in the shape of a serpent in the subtle body at the base of the spine. When awakened by appropriate Yoga practices, this "serpent" power uncoils and starts rising along the spine through the channel of the subtle body called *suṣumnā.* On its way it passes through six spiritual centres (*cakras*) and activates them, which results in the acquisition of special psychic powers on the part of the Yogi. The climax is reached when *Kuṇḍalinī* arrives at the top of the skull, which is the highest point of its journey but is no longer quite a part of the Yogi's subtle body. It represents a gate to Enlightenment and is referred to as the "thousand-petalled lotus" (*sahasrāra padma*). It seems that some Yoga schools believed that Enlightenment could be reached merely through the practice of Kuṇḍalinī Yoga, by compelling the passage of the *Kuṇḍalinī śakti* which represents also the creative spiritual force of the universe through the spiritual centres of the subtle body to the thousand-petalled lotus. However, the prevailing opinion seems to be that accompanying exercises of a spiritual kind are necessary. Spiritual Yoga, which nearly always follows Patañjali's scheme to some extent or other, is therefore, being superior, called *Rāja Yoga* or the "royal path".

As indicated, the spiritual energy (*śakti*) of *Kuṇḍalinī* is supposed to be essentially the same creative energy that, on the cosmic level, brings about the manifestation of the universe. In unawakened men this energy is responsible for their sexual and procreational potency. This being so, a view was developed that man's sexual energy could be directly utilised for the purpose of his spiritual progress. This is the province of *Tāntric Yoga*, a mysterious and as yet very little explored territory of Indian religious and Yogic tradition, despite the considerable amount of literature dealing with the subject. But it seems clear enough that Tāntrism in general and Tāntric Yoga in particular are split into two main schools of thought with corresponding Yoga practices. If the sexual energy is utilised directly for spiritual practice by being transformed into pure spiritual energy, one speaks about right-hand Tāntric practice. If sexual practices on the physical level are a part of the methodical procedure with the alleged aim of thereby inducing a direct experience of and link to the cosmic creative forces, it is left-hand Tāntric practice.[1]

1. Interest in Kuṇḍalinī Yoga and Tāntric teachings in the West started after the publication of the works of Arthur Avalon (Sir John Woodroffe). A vast literature on the subject has developed since, most of it unreliable or unusable so that the subject can still be regarded as little explored. It is dubious whether real light will ever be shed on Tāntrism through research, since Tāntric practice seems to have been transmitted directly from teacher to pupil and no Tāntric literary sources exist or have been discovered so far which would be comparable in reliability to those of other schools of Yoga and religious practice in India.

## Chapter VII

# YOGA IN THE MODERN WORLD

Yoga is and, as has been shown, has always been, in one form or another, an integral part of Indian civilisation. There were times when it was very much in the forefront, such as during the sixth and fifth centuries B. C., and there were other times when quite different phenomena dominated the scene of Indian history and life, such as during the eighteenth century, when the Mughal Empire was crumbling and the British were starting to step in, to become eventually the new rulers of the country and, more importantly, also the initiators of an encounter between two distinct cultures whose consequences have not yet been fully realized. But throughout the ages the living tradition of Yoga as an individual path to and a people's experience of the transcendent has been handed down from generation to generation till the present day.

As far as individuals are concerned, this handing down has been happening through the personal relationship between teachers and their pupils, some of whom themselves became teachers in turn, thus carrying on the tradition. On the national level the tradition has been kept alive by the deep regard for and veneration of Yogis and of "holy men" or spiritual truth-seekers on the part of all classes of Indian people. Besides, the old classical texts of Yoga have continued to be studied and commented on extensively, and new treatises on Yoga have been compiled from time to time.

During all these centuries many outstanding Yogis appeared on the scene. Some of them became famous in their own locality, some were renowned throughout India. Some (for example Śankara) made a name for themselves also in philosophy, and their teachings are subject even to academic research nowadays. Others were known only to their contemporaries and are survived by only a faint memory, and many must have been forgotten altogether.

The fact that Yoga and the lives of some Yogis have become the subject of study and academic research is, of course, due to the emergence of India as a part of the modern world after the arrival of British rule and, subsequently, the continuing pursuit by independent India of European-style learning. Further, the irresistible attraction of Western technology has changed life in India in the same way as anywhere else, especially in the field of communication. As a result of the publicity afforded them, events and personalities which in past ages might have remained of only local significance, have become known to and important for the whole country. This process has not stopped on the frontiers of India, and so the world now knows about the unbroken tradition of spiritual and religious search in India that is capable of producing saints even nowadays and thus offers an opportunity of exploring the mysterious regions of spiritual experience under the direct guidance of masters who claim authority in the field.

The Indians themselves soon became conscious of the Western world's interest in their spiritual tradition and quickly started adopting a Western-style approach to spreading its message abroad.

The first modern Indian saint to become world-famous was Ramakrishna and the first apostle of Indian spirituality in the West was his pupil, Vivekananda. It is worthwhile to sketch their lives briefly here.

Ramakrishna was born in 1836 in Kamarpukur, a small village in Bengal. His parents belonged to the caste of Brāhmans, but were quite poor. He was obviously a spiritually gifted child, for he had his first extraordinary experience when he was six years old. The beauty of a dark cloud and a flight of snow-white cranes produced an ecstasy in him while he was walking through the fields. He was so overwhelmed that he lost consciousness and was later brought home by a neighbour who had found him lying in a field. But he was also gifted intellectually and studied diligently the literature of Hinduism. Further more, he showed great talent for acting, which was always combined, in the traditional Indian style, with singing and dancing, and formed a theatre group to perform episodes from the Rāmāyaṇa and Mahābhārata. He was at his best when impersonating Kṛṣṇa, the human incarnation of the god Viṣṇu. Occasional ecstasies took possession of him while he was performing.

Another influence in his early life was his contact with pilgrims staying overnight in a nearby resthouse on their way to their destinations. He listened to their stories and religious conversations and sometimes even took part in them, showing great intelligence. When he was sixteen his elder brother, who ran a Sanskṛt College in Calcutta, invited him to join him and start a scholarly career, but Ramakrishna refused. By then he felt that all he was interested in was acquiring wisdom. He felt the urge to follow in the footsteps of many generations of Indian sages. But he did not become a homeless pilgrim, settling down instead as an appointed priest of a temple dedicated to the goddess Kālī in Dakshineshvar near Calcutta, in 1856.

In this subservient position he came in touch with crowds of devotees and watched the variegated expressions of their search for the Divine. Although at first not much attracted to it, the extraordinary atmosphere of the temple gradually absorbed him and he dedicated all his thoughts, prayers and meditations to Kālī, whose statue dominated the temple's interior.

Kālī represents in the Hindu Pantheon the mysterious force of nature that creates innumerable forms of life, but destroys, at the same time, so many of her creations. She is simultaneously the Divine Mother and the terrible destroyer of all things. Ramakrishna's duty as Kālī's priest was to perform all the rites prescribed in the daily routine of worship. But he soon became unable to carry out these duties, because he frequently either got lost in an ecstasy or started behaving as if he himself were the deity. But although numerous complaints started to be made about his erratic behaviour, no one, when face to face with him, dared to reprimand him. His sincerity, and the purity of his mind and character, were beyond doubt. Consequently, he was exempted from most of his duties and a year's leave was arranged for him so that he could live with his mother. During his stay at home he was married to a five year old girl (in 1859), later known as Sarada Devī, who, of course, returned to her home after the ceremony, according to the Hindu custom.

After his year's leave, with a somewhat recovered balance, Ramakrishna returned to his temple, but there his visions and ecstasies started with heightened intensity. This went so far that he began to suffer mentally as well as physically from the continuous strain. At that critical stage help from outside appeared, quite in keeping with the old Indian tradition, according to which a sincere truth-seeker finds help at the right moment. The help came in the form of a *saṅnyāsinī*, a homeless, female wanderer known as Bhairavī Brāhmaṇī.

This remarkable woman knew both the Hindu scriptures and the practical methods of Yoga, and what Ramakrishna had achieved on his own by the force of his devotion she helped him to go through again with full consciousness and in a disciplined way. Thus he realized consciously his oneness with God not only in the shape of Kālī, his Divine Mother, but also in whatever form he chose to approach him. He reached the summit of Bhakti Yoga and became widely recognised as one in whom God himself was revealed as in previous divine incarnations, such as that of Kṛṣṇa.

But this was not yet the end of the journey. After about three years he began to feel the mystery of the impersonal divine essence prowling round him. He did not like it, he shuddered to think what it meant—for it meant that he would have to give up, to renounce his cherished union with his Divine Mother or any other form of the Divine and to plunge into the mystery of the unmanifest.

As it transpired, he did not knowingly choose this path, but it chose him. In 1864 a naked ascetic known as Tota Puri arrived. He had the reputation of being an accomplished sage who had reached, after forty years of struggle, the lofty experience of the transcendent as described by the teachings of Advaita Vedānta. He never used to stay for more than three days in any one place. When he saw Ramakrishna, he told him : "My son, I see that you have already travelled far along the way of truth. If you wish it, I can help you to reach the next stage. I will teach you the Vedānta."[1]

Ramakrishna asked his Divine Mother for permission and when she agreed he submitted himself to the stranger's guidance. He had to renounce his cloth, his Brāhman's cord and his way of worship, together with his Bhakti affection for any form

1. See Rolland, *The Life of Ramakrishna*, p. 53.

or manifestation of the Divine. When he performed a symbolical burial rite signifying the death of his human ego, he was given the saffron robe of a sannyāsi. Then he received Advaitic instruction and in one day accomplished the goal of Jñāna Yoga, the *nirvikalpa saṅnyāsi*. Tota Puri was astonished and, having been Ramakrishna's teacher for a day, remained with him for eleven more months, more or less as his pupil, for Ramakrishna was able to convey to him the full validity of his previous realization of the Divine as the personal God.

Ramakrishna's spiritual position thereafter could be understood as one of reconciliation of the two seemingly opposite views of the highest reality. In its latency it is *Brahman*, the impersonal One. In its active aspect, it is the creative power known as *Śakti*, *Māyā* or *Prakṛti* and can be experienced as the personal God. But this distinction does not, in fact, represent a real difference. *Brahman* and the Divine Mother are one.

When Tota Puri left, Ramakrishna spent six months in *samādhi*, almost without interruption, hardly prepared to return to life. But the bodily suffering with which his organism reacted to his neglect brought him back to everyday consciousness. When he recovered, he was a new man, balanced and integrated and conscious of his mission, which was to teach others, to spread the message of spiritual life. People of all kinds and shades of Hindu belief poured to him. But he realized that spirituality was not limited to Hinduism as its channel. Indeed, there were more paths to it even within Hinduism itself, as his own experience had shown. As the different deities of Hinduism were manifestations of one and the same highest reality, so were the gods of different religions. When seeing a Muslim (Govinda Rai) in deep prayer, he realized that this man also had found God. He asked him for initiation and instruction and lived then as a Muslim for some time. This resulted in visions of Mohammad followed by the experience of universal oneness (1866). Some years later (1874) a friend read the Bible to him. Soon after that Ramakrishna had visions of the Madonna and Jesus and later on of Christ. They were much more intense than his Islamic visions and for some time he was pervaded by the spirit of Christ to the exclusion of everything else. But even these experiences finally merged with the realization of the absolute. After that, Christ, along with Kṛṣṇa and the Buddha, was a real incarnation of God for him.

In the meantime Sarada Devi, Ramakrishna's wife, came to join him. She became his pupil, while at the same time he looked on her, as on every woman, as an incarnation of his Divine Mother, Kālī. Their marriage remained always a purely spiritual partnership, and Sarada Devi looked after him and the growing circle of his disciples.

Ramakrishna was becoming more and more famous. Nobody doubted his high achievements, and his power to transform others was enormous. Ordinary people and educated individuals, Indians and visitors from abroad, all felt the strong presence of spirituality in him. When he died in 1886 a group of his closest pupils formed a monastic community under the leadership of Vivekananda. Later the movement grew into a world-wide organisation, the "Ramakrishna Math Mission" which still exists.[1]

1. There is abundant literature on Ramakrishna, his life, sayings and conversations. One of the first tributes was paid to him by no less a man than Max Müller. Perhaps the first article that made Ramakrishna known in the West was by Prof. C.H. Tawney, A Modern Hindu Saint" in the *Imperial and Quarterly Review*, January 1896. Then came Max Müller's "A Real Mahatma" in the *Nineteenth Century* of 1896, where Prof. Müller confronted the real living saint of India, Ramakrishna, with the imaginary Mahatmas of the Theosophical Society. Later came the book : M. Müller : *Ramakrishna, His Life and Sayings*, London 1896 (last published in 1923).

One work which contributed very much to the fame of Ramakrishna and was translated into several languages was written by the well-known French author Romain Rolland under the title *Ramakrishna the Man-God and the Universal Gospel of Vivekananda. A Study of Mysticism and Action in Living India* (1929).

It is now available in two volumes printed in India:

R. Rolland : *The Life of Ramakrishna*, Calcutta 1965.

,, *The Life of Vivekananda*, Almora 1944.

A good contemporary presentation of Ramakrishna's life and teaching, including post-history of the movement, is given by the following book :

S. Lemaitre : *Ramakrishna et la vitalite de l'hindouisme*. Paris 1959.

Vivekananda is the second great name connected with the spreading of knowledge about Yoga in modern times. His intelligence and intellectual capacity made him an able apostle of Ramakrishna's teaching to the West. He was born in 1863 in Calcutta in an aristocratic (*kṣatriya*) family. He was an undergraduate when he first visited Ramakrishna and was told by him straightaway that he had been chosen to continue his mission. After some initial mistrust and inner struggles he succumbed to Ramakrishna's charm and spiritual influence. Eventually he was helped by him to achieve even the highest samādhi experience.

After his master's death and when he had consolidated the newly founded monastic order, Vivekananda spent some time in solitude in the Himalaya, and then travelled India for two years spreading Ramakrishna's Gospel. In 1893 he left for the USA via China and Japan to take part in the "Parliament of Religions" in Chicago where he became "undoubtedly the greatest figure".[1] Following up his success in the Parliament, he toured the States lecturing and taking classes. In subsequent years he visited Europe and found many admirers and pupils, especially in England. He returned to India a national hero after four years of travel. He reorganised the small community of *saṅnyāsis* as a result of his new experiences and soon Vedānta centres were founded in other parts of India and in Western countries. Thus the Ramakrishna Mission was set in motion. During the years 1899-1900 Vivekananda undertook his second journey to the West to inspect and consolidate the results of his work. He visited England, spent a year in the USA and a few months in France. Back at home, he died in 1902.

Vivekananda was a great Advaita Vedāntist and Jñāna Yogi and it was owing to him that Indian philosophy and Yoga began to fire the imagination of many people in Western countries as early as the end of the last century. Prompted by the urging of his master Ramakrishna and helped by the historical situation of India, which was responsible for his English education, Vivekananda started a trend for popularity of Yoga, which, with inevitable ups and downs, has stayed with us ever since.

In a way he was also responsible for the still widely held popular misconception of Yoga as being an "Eastern philosophy"

1. The New York Herald. See Rolland, *Life of Vivekananda*, p. 44.

and also for the general impression, still persisting in the minds of many Westerners, that the basis of Indian philosophical speculation and Yoga realization is the illusoriness of the world and the sole reality of *Brahman*. But this, of course, is merely the most extreme interpretation of the Advaita Vedānta school of philosophy which Vivekanda appears to have followed in some respects. Other philosophical conceptions have been discussed in this book and one of its objectives is to show that Yoga cannot, in fact, be correctly identified with any of them.

Both Ramakrishna and Vivekananda belonged to the last century, although their influence can still be felt. Let us now turn to two other great Yogis of India who lived mainly and were active as Yogis solely in this century and who both became world-famous. They were Ramaṇa Maharṣi of Arunachala and Aurobindo Ghosh.

Ramaṇa was born on the 30th of December 1879 in Tiruchizhi in South India of a Brāhman family. While receiving high school education he did not show any signs of being exceptional, but suddenly in June 1896 he went through an unusual experience. For no obvious reason a violent fear of death came upon him. He felt sure he would die just then. Without much thought he accepted the fact and lay down, ready to watch what would happen after the body died. Suddenly he realized that thus watching his body and expecting its processes to come to an end, he himself was not at all the same as his body and that this "I" of his was, in fact, the spiritual Self independent of the body and unable to die. His fear of death disappeared and he did not die physically, but he was never the same again. The realization of the higher Self remained with him ever afterwards.

For a few subsequent weeks he lived or tried to live as before, going to school and living at home. But it did not work. There was no motivation in him to pursue the activities of an ordinary life. Consequently, he left home secretly and made his way to Tiruvannamalai at the foot of the hill Arunachala, which had the reputation of being a holy place and which attracted him. There he stayed, sitting absorbed in deep meditation and caring for nothing, within the precincts of the temple, mostly in an underground pit to escape the attention of the public. Later he moved around from time to time. His austere way of life gained him recognition and so there was always someone to look after his very limited needs.

Ramaṇa did not speak or communicate with anybody in any way for about three years. But people were drawn to him constantly and were satisfied with a "*darśan*" of him (just to come and see him). He seemed to live mostly in deep meditative absorption, but eventually he was moved by the eager questions of some visitors and started answering questions by scribbling on small slips of paper. These slips, put together, represent the manuscripts of his two small works that were published later—"Self Enquiry" and "Who Am I?". Subsequently he wrote some poems or songs of devotion and these were frequently sung by *sādhus* (mendicants) staying with him. Finally he began to talk and many of his conversations were recorded. A few further writings and translations of older Sanskṛt works originated as instructions to the pupils now gathered round him. His reputation as an accomplished master steadily grew and so did the stream of visitors from all over India and finally also from abroad. Many of these visitors recorded afterwards that they had forgotten their prepared questions in his presence and had experienced profound peace or bliss or a kind of illumination instead.

Ramaṇa remained at Arunachala until he died on the 4th of April 1950. He had become known all over the world. Even outstanding politicians visited him, among them were the two late Presidents of India, Dr. Rajendra Prasad and Professor S. Radhakrishnan. Even those visitors who came more out of curiosity than to receive help in some earnest search for spiritual guidance were most impressed by him. But many people considered themselves to be his pupils on the path of Yoga and many seem to follow his method even nowadays. He did not bring any new teaching or philosophy and he might be described as fitting within the tradition of Advaita Vedānta. Neither is his method new. His insrtuctions especially the two books mentioned above, can be classified as following the path of Jñāna Yoga. But they are formulated so as to be easily understood today. They offer a method of self-inquiry that is basically analytical and proceeds, first discursively and then meditationally, to eliminate the meditator's identification with insubstantial constituents of his personality—which are his body, his feelings and his thoughts—

in order to enable him to penetrate to the experience of his hidden essence or "real self".[1]

Aurobindo Ghosh represents an entirely different type of Yogi from Ramaṇa. This is already reflected in his early life and education. He was born on the 15th of August 1872 in Calcutta. His father was a westernised intellectual, a doctor by profession, who saw to it that his children got a European education. Aurobindo was sent at the age of five to a convent school in Darjeeling and two years later to England where he was first educated privately. Then after two years he entered St. Paul's school in West Kensington. He was an excellent pupil and, having received a grant, entered King's College, Cambridge. Extremely successful in his Classical Tripos, he did not qualify for the Civil Service (for which his father had intended him) only because he failed to pass the horse-riding examination then prescribed for that career. This may have been an outcome consciously or unconsciously wished for, as Aurobindo was not at all attracted to the Civil Service, but he would not directly oppose his father's wish. Besides, life in England had awakened in him an interest in his own country and her destiny

1. The first knowledge about Ramaṇa Maharṣi was transmitted to Western readers by the book : P. Brunton : *A Search in Secret India*, London 1934.

It was this book that was chiefly responsible for the subsequent constant flow of visitors from Western countries to Ramaṇa's *āśram*. Among them was also the distinguished German traveller Veltheim-Ostrau referred to earlier. As happened in the case of Ramakrishna, Ramaṇa Maharṣi was also paid a tribute by an indologist of outstanding quality.

H. Zimmer : *Der Weg zum Selbst : Leben und Lehre des indischen Heiligen Shri Ramana Maharshi aus Tiruvannamalei. Mit einem Vorwort hrsg. von C. G. Jung*. Neuausgabe, Zurich 1954.

An authentic account of Ramaṇa's influence on a Western pupil of his who became an Indian mendicant is given in the autobiographical book :

Mouni Sadhu : *In Days of Great Peace*, London 1952.

A useful biography was issued by the *Āśram* as its official publication : *Śri Maharshi. A Short Life Sketch*. Tiruvannamalai 1963 (4th ed.).

Ramaṇa's own works and translations form a small book : *The Collected Works of Ramaṇa Maharshi*. Edited and annotated by A. Osborne, London 1959

and he became, step by step, an Indian nationalist committed to fight for India's independence.

In 1893 Aurobindo returned home and entered the service of the Mahārāja of Baroda, first in the State Department, later as teacher of English and English literature at Baroda College of which he eventually became Principal. In 1906 he was offered the post of Principal of the National College in Calcutta. In 1901 he had married, but his subsequent political and later spiritual pursuits led to long periods of separation from his wife that stood in the way of their mutual understanding. Besides, the marriage had been pre-arranged according to Indian custom, his wife was fifteen years younger than he and, although she tried to some extent to understand or even follow his interests, she was not of the stature to succeed. She died in 1918 while still quite young.

Soon after his return to India Aurobindo started to be interested in Yoga. But he embarked on studying it not for its proclaimed goal, but because it was supposed to give power and he wanted power in order to use it in politics. He started practising seriously in 1904, doing *prāṇāyāma* exercises for five hours a day. He later wrote that he had had extremely good results. He felt he had acquired heightened energy and mental efficiency and decided to seek expert guidance in order to progress further. He got in touch with a Yoga Guru called Vishnu Bhaskar Lele who instructed him in meditation—how to control the mind and keep it free from intruding thoughts. Within three days of commencing secluded meditations with the Guru, Aurobindo reached a state of inner stillness that remained with him ever after, as he later wrote. This happened in December 1907. Aurobindo went further in his meditations and achievement than his Guru had anticipated. He could not teach him further, and gave him the advice to listen to and follow the guru within himself.

This new dimension of inner experience had a profound influence on Aurobindo; it had more reality for him than the outside world with all its events. It also fitted well with the Vedāntic view of the world process as being a sequence of empty forms against the background of the absolute and impersonal *Brahman*. Aurobindo felt from that time on that he was a free spiritual being. But he also felt that there was still more to come, that he was not yet at the end of the road.

By this time, however, he was also deeply involved in revolutionary political activities aimed at India's full political independence. He was the editor of *Bande Mātaram*, a revolutionary magazine, and belonged to a secret revolutionary organization whose training included combat, riding, shooting and also home-made bomb testing. Now he did not know what to do. But the solution came without his active decision. In May 1908 the British Government of India made a move against radical and revolutionary activities and rounded up about a hundred leaders. Aurobindo was one of them and he spent a year in the solitude of Alipur prison awaiting trial. That year became a turning-point in his life. He spent most of the time doing Yoga exercises and meditating. His experience of the spiritual dimension deepened and changed into what Aurobindo later called communication with the Divine Mind. He received direct guidance from this source both as to his immediate situation and for his long-term future. After a year he was released from prison and his first public appearance was a speech in Uttapara which was wholly and purely religious.

One cannot be surprised that the authorities did not readily accept his conversion as a genuine. When warned that he might be arrested again, he published his political testament. In it he again stressed the inevitability of India's complete independence and the right of her people to shape their lives freely according to their tradition and character. But he added that this goal did not include hate against any other nation, not even against the present government. The ideal of India's independence presupposed the unity of her people and this in turn was an anticipation of the future unity of mankind. The means used to achieve independence should remain within the boundaries of the law.

To escape the danger of arrest Aurobindo left Calcutta and finally, driven by the insistence of his inner vocation, he settled down in the French colony of Pondicherry, in April 1910. That was the end of his political career, but a new one started for him and lasted for the rest of his life, which ended on the

5th December 1950. It was the life of a Yogi, a philosopher and a Guru.

The beginnings of his new life were quite difficult and it took several years before Aurobindo became established. Four friends from his revolutionary period accompanied him as his first pupils in Yoga and the circle started slowly but steadily to grow. An important factor in this process became the magazine *Ārya* which Aurobindo started in 1914. The idea came from Paul Richard, a French civil servant who was very impressed by Aurobindo. Many later philosophical works were published in their original version in this magazine, which soon gained an international reputation and brought new pupils to what was now becoming an *Āśram.*

In 1920 Aurobindo was joined by Mira Richard who soon became the "Mother" of the *Āśram.* Born in Egypt of a Turkish family with some Jewish connections, she was married to Paul Richard and so met Aurobindo in 1914. She had studied religious and occult literature and had even been trained by an "occult Master" in Algeria. On meeting Aurobindo she immediately felt that he was her real Master. The war removed her and her husband from Pondicherry, but she returned as soon as she could, this time alone. At first she took charge of running the *Āśram's* practical affairs, but the feeling of congeniality must have been mutual, for in 1926 Aurobindo entrusted her with the full leadership of the *Āśram* and withdrew into solitude. His pupils could reach him only by writing or through the mediation of the Mother. Only on special occasions did he show himself to his pupils, devotees, and visitors. The Mother headed the *Āśram* till her death in 1973. It has grown over the years into a modern establishment with many facilities and in addition a whole new city for 50,000 inhabitants—Auroville—is under construction (with the support of well-wishers from all over the world and of UNESCO). The community will live there according to the principles of Aurobindo's philosophy.

This philosophy is one of spiritual evolutionism. Aurobindo appreciates the evolution one can see in the world (as expressed in Western sciences, particularly after Darwin), but he sees behind it the Divine Mind at work. When, however, evolution produces man, it does not automatically continue further. From then on it is man's task to bring about further progress in himself and in the world by consciously securing the help of the Divine Mind, which otherwise would not work for his progress. By his efforts man becomes a collaborator with the Divine Mind in the work of spiritualising the Universe (see chapter IV). The individual way to such collaboration with the Divine Mind is Integral Yoga.

Integral Yoga is Aurobindo's answer to the fragmentation of Yoga that it has suffered since its classical period (roughly speaking after Śankara). It would be futile to try to characterise it briefly, but it is possible to say that it seems to incorporate the classical Yoga methods as known from Patañjali and the Buddhist eightfold path as well as the broad and universal outlook of the *Bodhisattva* ideal as developed in Mahāyāna Buddhism. The latter is reflected in Aurobindo's concern for the redemption of the whole universe. But Aurobindo's inspiration is drawn also from much older sources, particularly the Vedic hymns. On the other hand, the deep influence of the Bhagavad Gītā is also traceable.

Aurobindo has made Yoga and the Indian type of spiritual philosophy presentable and even palatable to Western academic circles. At the same time he has found a following among people of all classes all over the world. His universalism made him also into a leading figure in humanity's struggle for a future cultural synthesis.[1]

Almost simultaneously with the remarkable modern revival of Hinduism and with Yoga's achievement of world-wide popularity, there occurred also the revival of Buddhism and the Buddhist methods of meditation which are only seldom referred to as Buddhist Yoga, although there is no reason why this term should not be employed. But no illustrious names mark this revival as they do in the case of Hinduism, for Buddhism does not favour the image of spiritual teachers. The Buddhist train-

1. For Aurobindo's life the most important source is the work *Sri Aurobindo on Himself* and *The Mother*, contained in the first volume of the Pondicherry edition of his works.

There are many books on Aurobindo's life and teachings that have varying degrees of usefulness. One of the more useful ones is the following :

*Sri Aurobindo in Selbstzeugnissen und Bilddokumenten.* Dargestellt von. O Wolff. Rowohlt 1967.

ing usually takes place in monastic establishments dating from earlier centuries and not in *āśramas* created around a famous guru. The person of a teacher, although important in the process of instruction and supervision, is not viewed as being the central force of spiritual influence.

Buddhism also was represented at the Chicago Parliament of Religions and its speaker there was Anagarika Dharmapala from Ceylon. He represented the Theravāda school of Buddhism, whose scriptural basis is the Pāli Canon and its commentaries, and had a considerable success. Knowledge of Buddhism had been spread until then by the works of scholars, but popular literature also started appearing at that time and in ever increasing quantity afterwards.

Buddhism originally appealed to the Western mind chiefly on account of the rational elements in its teachings and also the global systematic framework of its spiritual practice which required no specifically religious approach nor any belief in dogmas. Its practical core could be easily established. As a result, as early as in the 1880's a number of Western people joined monastic communities in Asia, mainly in Ceylon, in order to practise the Buddhist path. In the early years of this century a community of European Buddhist monks, which still exists, was created on Dondaduwa, a little island off Ceylon. Its founder was Nyānatiloka Mahāthera, a German by birth, who became known as a writer on Buddhism and a translator of Buddhist texts. Another outstanding representative of the European monkhood in Ceylon is Nyāṇaponika Thera of the Forest Hermitage near Kandy, who is also of German origin.

It seems that real spiritual practice in the Buddhist monasteries had been largely neglected for some centuries, and in its place the study of original Pāli texts and commentaries and an attitude of worship had prevailed. A wider revival of interest in the effort to practise meditations seems to have come from Burma at the beginning of this century when a monk, U Narada, following the instruction of an unnamed monk living in the hills of Upper Burma, set his mind to working out a method of meditation based on the texts dealing with *satipaṭṭhāna* or the "establishing of mindfulness". His success led to his becoming a teacher of others and when he died in 1955 he had the reputation (which is never much emphasised in Buddhist circles) of being a saint.

The renewed interest in *satipaṭṭhāna* meditation spread to other Buddhist countries, such as Thailand and Ceylon and, in the course of time, special meditation centres were created for strict meditational practice under the supervision of experienced teachers. They are usually open to both monks and laymen who spend limited periods under training there in order to be able to continue the practice on their own. The *satipaṭṭhāna* method taught in these centres is described as meditational training in "insight" (*vipassanā bhāvanā*) and is based mainly on the elaboration of the seventh part of the Buddhist eightfold path (*sammā sati* or right mindfulness).

The method of meditation that leads to the development of absorptions (*samatha bhāvanā*) does not seem to be favoured by present-day Buddhist meditation teachers. It is seen as little suited for the present conditions prevailing in the world, in the West as well as in the East, at least in the initial stages of the path.[1] Buddhist meditation has also become attractive and popular in Western countries in its Japanese Zen form, which is, however, outside the scope of this work.

Whoever has studied Yoga literature, whether ancient or modern or both, cannot but be impressed by the extraordinary vitality of Yoga, the variety of its forms, its undeniable achievements, and the multitude of possible ways and levels of approach to its goal. Behind all this variety the final aim of Yoga appears always to be one, namely a state of final liberation or salvation, however variedly defined, which is in turn, it is sometimes claimed, identical with the goal of all higher religions despite their differing ideas or conceptions of it.

Another interesting feature of Yoga is the fact that some phenomena produced in the course of its practice, both in the physiology of the human body and in the psychology of the human

1. Literature on the revival of interest in Buddhist meditational practices is centred much less round personal biographies and life stories of teachers than is the case with the revival of the Hindu type Yoga. An interesting account of personal experience in Burmese meditation centres is given in the book :

M.B. Byles : *Journey into Burmese Silence*, London 1962.

personality, attract the attention of some scientists. But by far the most conspicuous impact of Yoga in the West is its appeal to a vast number of people who take up some moderate form of Yoga practice and introduce it into their daily lives, because they feel that it fills a gap in the pattern of their existence.

We can describe the impact of Yoga on the Western mind as having three aspects; popular, scientific and religious-philosophical. But naturally they are not quite separate and overlap each other to a considerable extent.

The popular appeal of Yoga in the West is concentrated mainly around its physical form, called Haṭha Yoga. This is in keeping with the prevailing preoccupation of masses of people with tangible and everyday values of life. Thus Haṭha Yoga is frequently treated and presented as a "health and beauty" device. Indian texts on Haṭha Yoga[1] claim fantastic-sounding benefits that supposedly result from the practice of various positions (*āsanas*). In a weakened or watered down form, promises or indications of benefits to health as a result of regular practice of the *āsanas* are incorporated in all popular books on and text books of Haṭha Yoga.

These claims sometimes have medical backing, although this may be only conditional, based as it is so far on insufficient research and limited experience.[2] But there are few, if any, members of the medical profession nowadays who are not prepared to recognise some benefits stemming from regular Haṭha Yoga practice carried out moderately or with competence. And regularly practised Haṭha Yoga exercises do, no doubt, have a profound influence on the fitness of a number of the constituents of the human organism.

Firstly there is their influence on preserving or even increasing the flexibility of the spine and the joints, which is quite important in the context of modern living which has brought too much comfort and requires too little movement. Secondly, all the *āsanas* exercise a deep influence on the blood circulation; some of the positions bring blood to parts and organs of the body that otherwise never get such an abundant supply all at once:

1. *Gheraṇḍa Saṁhita*, *Śiva Saṁhitā* and *Haṭha Yoga Pradīpikā*.
2. See Dr. G.J. Mukerji and Dr. W. Spiegelhoff : *Yoga und unsere Medizin*, Stuttgart 1963.

other parts are relieved from an oversupply of blood, and some positions even cause the blood to be squeezed out of a particular organ for a moment, only to allow it to return in a flushing wave. These procedures obviously enhance the distribution of oxygen and nourishment to various parts of the organism, and the removal of toxic and dead materials.

Thirdly, there are exercises that influence the digestive organs by a kind of internal massage; the results in terms of bodily freshness, rejuvenation and improved external appearance are not only the subjective feelings of the trainees. Fourthly, there is an undoubted powerful, although subtle, influence from the Haṭha Yoga exercises on the nervous system. Some positions obviously squeeze certain nerves and create pressures in some nerve centres thereby obtaining a stimulating result without the after-effects produced by chemical stimulants. In addition, Haṭha Yoga also teaches a special technique of relaxation that affects all the systems of the body, including the nervous system, as well as the mind.

All these effects justify the popularity of Haṭha Yoga and stress its usefulness in the context of modern living as one of a variety of possible means that man can choose in order to make his way of life healthier and more balanced. Thousands of Yoga courses are organised in many Western countries. In Great Britain most of them are run nowadays under the auspices of local authorities in their adult education establishments. But there is also a number of private Yoga teachers and centres as well as a national organisation called the Wheel of Yoga.[1]

1. The level on which Haṭha Yoga is taught in the West is fairly elementary, but generally speaking it seems to be quite competent and adequate to the purpose. There is an abundance of Haṭha Yoga textbooks. One of the earliest propagators of Haṭha Yoga in Europe was S. Yesudian who came to Budapest in the 1930's and started a Yoga school. Later he moved to Switzerland. His book *Sport und Yoga* (Thielle 1949), translated into English as *Yoga and Health* (London 1953) gives a basic sequence of *āsanas* which practically everybody can master and which are also described in almost all other books on the subject. At the other end of the scale we meet with the comprehensive approach of B. K. S. Iyenger (who counts among his disciples some illustrious personages, such as Yehudi Menuhin and the Belgian Queen Mother) whose book *Light on Yoga* (London 1965) describes over 230 *āsanas* many of them extremely difficult, to be mastered only after years of dedicated practice and only if started at a young age.

While the tide of Yoga's popularisation in the West is running high, its impact on the scientific scene is hardly noticeable. But that does not mean that it is absent, only that it has not yet come fully to light. There are many individual therapists and also clinics utilising Yoga methods, sometimes in a modified form, for physical rehabilitation, for treatment of various ailments, for psychotherapy and also for the prevention of physical as well as mental ill-health. Both the physical and mental aspects of Yoga are involved.[1] Some basic scientific research has also already been done into the measurable physiological and psychological results of Haṭha Yoga exercises, relaxation and mental Yoga techniques.[2] But it is still in its very beginnings and much more work will be required before Yoga as a special branch of "science of man" will be generally recognised or established in some form in the West. However, there is now much more open-mindedness and much less scepticism forthcoming from scientific quarters than a decade or two ago with respect to the unexplored possibilities of the human organism and psyche that Yoga seems to be capable of opening up.

The impact of Yoga on the Western mind in the sphere of religious and philosophical thinking is not very conspicuous, either. But again, it undoubtedly has had some impact, and it is likely to keep increasing. The ways in which Yoga exercises some influence have been mostly indirect, through Indian philosophical thinking. If we disregard the possible early influence of Indian teachings on ancient neo-Platonism, the first undoubted traces of fascination that Indian thought exercised on some Western philosophers can be found in A. Schopenhauer. Hegel and other German idealists like Schlegel and Fichte would, on analysis, reveal that they, too, had not altogether escaped the influence. In America, transcendentalism,

1. These activities also go on in India where they sometimes take the form of combined research institutes with hospitals attached. Yoga-therapy is applied under conditions that are up to Western medical standard and most members of the staff have appropriate medical training, perhaps the most important institute of this type is in Lonavla. Another, perhaps more modest, is in Santa Cruz, Bombay.

2. See some contributions in the previously quoted book, *Forms And Techniques of Altruistic And Spiritual Growth.*

represented mainly by R.W. Emerson, is a clear example of Indian influence. In England the work of F.H. Bradley might merit investigation along these lines.

During the last two or three decades, which—apart from existentialism—have seen few, if any, new developments in philosophising, it has been the fairly new academic discipline called Comparative Philosophy that has brought Indian philosophical and religious ideas to the forum of philosophical discussion. Similarly, Comparative Religion, whose importance is being more and more recognised, directs much attention to Indian religious phenomena.[1] In both these disciplines Yoga receives due attention. Besides, it may again be pointed out in this context that the creative stimulus for much of the philosophical and religious thought in India can be traced to a source that is nourished by insights gained through some kind of Yoga involvement. This was true in the past (as in the case of the Upaniṣadic philosophy, and of the philosophy of Buddhism and of Vedānta) and it is also happening in the present time (as in the case of Aurobindo).

It is still too early to try to see specific signs of the influence of the new comparative approach in original philosophical work. But on a broader basis some influence is quite obvious, particularly on the religious front. In the first place it is seen in the interest mentioned earlier of some Christian representatives and believers in using Yoga meditational techniques to bring new depth into their experience of Christianity.[2] This is

1. Both disciplines have already extensive literature to their credit. There seem to be no systematic guides to their study. Therefore it is necessary to start with some introductory works and follow up references given in them. E.g. :

P. T. Raju : *Introduction to Comparative Philosophy*, Lincoln (USA) (1962.

J. Wach : *The Comparative Study of Religions*, New York 1958.

2. When it sometimes appears, especially in Germany, that it is Zen meditation rather than the traditional Indian Yoga that is being explored for the possible help it can provide for Christians, this nonetheless supports the case of the influence of Yoga, Zen meditation being a Buddhist Yoga technique quite in line with and in the last instance based on the Buddhist eightfold path, particularly its seventh and eighth parts.

in a way a recognition of the fact that the sources of inner spiritual experience once present within Christianity as living mysticism are no longer or are insufficiently alive, whilst their vitality in the East is such that they can be drawn on, as it were, to revive the sources in the West and at the same time be expected to manifest themselves in a form congenial to the specific Christian belief.

But there is a second and perhaps potentially more important aspect of, and prospect for, this influence. A number, albeit probably a very small one, of the students of Yoga in the West is trying to put to practical test the claim of Yoga that it can, by the application of its techniques of mental training, develop spiritual experiences that transcend the normal capabilities of the mind. These people could not, perhaps, be called religious or religious-minded in the current sense of the word, but they are certainly interested in the effects of Yoga practice on more than just their health, their capacity to relax and perhaps some degree of peace of mind. They might be called "truth-seekers" and their philosophical or religious outlook does not include a firm commitment to any particular tradition. Yoga attracts them because its techniques, as derived from the systems of the Buddha and Patañjali, promise specific results in terms of the expansion of human knowledge into the dimension of spirituality, without committing them to any particular belief or philosophy, whether Hindu, Buddhist or otherwise.

This can be viewed as a very important development which might eventually lead to a break-through from the undoubted impasse in which the Western mind finds itself at present. The Western civilisation as it has developed is secular and very much science-orientated. Its secularity is a result of the advance of the sciences and of science-based technological progress. The Western civilisation was not always secular, it was Christian for a long time. One of the reasons, if not the main cause, for its secularisation was the failure of Christianity, at the dawn of the modern time, to keep pace with or even to grasp the unprecedented achievements of the human intellect in its inquiry into the working of reality as accessible to man's normal cognitive and reasoning capacities, and in its application of the newly gained knowledge in everyday life. The human intellect became fascinated by its own achievements and ceased to appreciate the deeper spiritual message of Christianity, buried under the outdated dogmatic formulations of a bygone era. The result was an overoptimistic belief that not only external nature, but also specifically human problems, like those of education, social behaviour and the harmony of communal life as well as those of individual happiness and personal integrity, could be regulated satisfactorily once enough scientific knowledge has been accumulated. But this attitude has proved self-defeating. The successes of science and technology, and particularly the enormous rise in the standard of living of the mass of the Western population, promoted with some a conscious acceptance and with others an unconscious and tacit adoption of a utilitarian and materialistic philosophy of life that is not conducive to foresight and has therefore led to crises that seem to be getting worse each time they occur and that cast the shadow of a possible general collapse of the whole civilisation.

Perhaps this is already enough to show that the progress of the sciences and of purely intellectual, rational knowledge, however admirable and desirable, cannot bring about progress in the sphere of specifically human affairs. Their outcome depends on the stage of man's spiritual development. This used to be the province of religion and, sometimes, of philosophy, if it aspired to spiritual insights (as for example with Pythagoras, Plato, Plotinos or Emerson). Can they still help nowadays?

Let us turn first to philosophy. What is its state and what are its aims? Modern philosophy appears to be highly fragmented into specialised disciplines, and of these logic and semantics or linguistic philosophy are in the forefront, particularly in this country. The aim of philosophers seems to be to emulate science and produce specialised answers to specialised questions in particular fields of intellectual interest, but without the chance or even the ambition to influence men's lives. It is as though philosophy has abdicated from its ancient task to look for the meaning of life.[1] There are a few, for instance K. Jaspers, who can bring their philosophical inquiry to the point at which they are faced with the unknown territory of transcen-

1. Cf. F.A. Lea : *A Defence of Philosophy*, London 1962.

dence and can see the necessity, at least as individuals, to seek further means of knowledge. True, there is also the phenomenological approach mentioned previously (see chapter I). But neither Husserl nor those who continue to work on the phenomenological method have produced sufficient results. Besides, both these approaches are so academic that their impact on the Western mind in general has so far been minimal.

Can Christianity, the religion of the West, offer modern man the way to the missing experience of spiritual values after all? Obviously Christianity is, in its various existing forms, aware of the problem and is trying to step in. Yet it seems that it is too late for it to catch up with the modern way of thinking and present its original message to man in some kind of present-day idiom. Indeed, it is questionable whether there is a modern Christian equivalent of the depth of spiritual experience which for mediaeval Christianity was represented by its living mysticism. Christianity as it has developed seems to be based too much on the requirement of belief in certain revelations that to a thinking mind appear to be historically conditioned symbols of a hidden spiritual reality, but are insisted on, within the Christian teachings, as being unique and factual events with universal and monopolistic spiritual validity. Without this belief there can hardly be any chance of reviving the deeper, mystical approach that alone can be satisfying in producing solutions to the problems of existence. If this way can still be followed, it will be open to only very few. But the modern Western civilisation as a whole has long been out of touch with and actually has grown more or less in conflict with or in opposition to traditional Christianity. There seems therefore to be no chance of a living mutual relationship developing between them.

The modern Western mind has become what it is through the adventures of its scientific discoveries. In the process it has developed its sharp and logically-working intellect as its most precious and effective tool for dealing with reality. There is nothing wrong with it or with the resulting technological civilisation in itself. Indeed, both the intellectual brilliance and the technological efficiency of the Western mind are high achievements now being emulated all over the world. But what the modern Western mind does lack is a certain dimension of depth that may best be called spirituality. Intellectual planning and technological ingenuity have changed man's life, made it easier, more comfortable, and up to a point more dignified. But they could not, in themselves, create the conditions for a sense of fulfilment in life. Further scientific discoveries and better planning of the environment will not provide the answer; they will never penetrate to the fundamental, deep issues of man's existence and its meaning which were provided for in the past by religion.

Yet the discovery or achievement of the link to this dimension of depth—to spirituality—cannot be something entirely different from, let alone contrary or contradictory to, the scientific approach to new knowledge. The high standards of the scientific method of research must have an equivalent in the quest for the dimension of depth in human life. And already some start has been made in this direction. Psychoanalysis and various subsequent schools of depth psychology have been developing their techniques for studying the inner dimensions of man's mind that are normally hidden from his everyday consciousness. The practical application of depth psychology is psychotherapy, in a somewhat similar way as technology is for science, but it is, of course, concerned only with adapting disturbed individuals to current conditions of life, and is not a search for a new and deeper integration of the human personality—although some authors do suggest that psychotherapy based on depth psychology opens the wider question of man's higher integration.[1]

1. S. Freud was already interested in the point, although mainly on a more general basis as is shown by his interest in "cultural psychoanalysis". And so was C.G. Jung, whose involvement in the study of religions, including Oriental ones, brought this point out more clearly and influenced subsequent psychoanalysts of all schools. One of them is E. Fromm, who is deeply preoccupied with the questions of man's integration, not only adaptation. The question is fully, though not perhaps very deeply, dealt with in the book :

A. Reza Arasteh : *Final Integration in the Adult Personality*, Leyden 1965.

Recently the British psychiatrist R. D. Laing has become preoccupied with this question.

And this is where Yoga may come in. No matter how quickly or how slowly depth psychology may be able to cope with this question, Yoga is already here as a developed, systematic way of exploring the inner dimensions of man's mind, a method of self-knowledge as well as of approach to the task of higher integration or the final maturing of the human personality in a way congenial to the intellectual standards required by the scientifically-trained mind. At the same time Yoga offers practical guidance also to non-specialists, that is to say to the ordinary man in the street who feels he needs to do something for himself yet cannot find or accept help from religion and cannot wait until depth psychology develops its own method and makes it available on a broad basis.

With respect to the last point, Yoga has already started to fulfil this task for a large and growing number of people, but one matter still needs to be mentioned in this context. The image of Yoga as such has to be kept separate from Hindu religious movements that are trying to missionise all over the world, such as the "International Society for Kṛṣṇa Consciousness Ltd.", or various organisations of proselytising Eastern gurus, for example the "Divine Light Society" headed by the teenage "perfect master" styled Guru Maharaj Ji. Generally speaking, there is nothing objectionable in movements like these, and they may be very useful to those who otherwise would not find any affiliation to religious or spiritual values, and they are certainly most interesting phenomena on the scene of contemporary religious development. But it has been the objective throughout this work to show that Yoga has to be understood in its own right and must not be mistaken for a cult or sectarian movement despite the fact that cults and sects make use of some of its methods and also use its terminology.

At the same time it has to be stressed again that, in the last instance, Yoga does reach into the spheres that have traditionally been the domain of religions and of philosophy or metaphysics. And it is here that it has its particular significance also for the average Western man in the street. His education, even where it was minimal and formally finished at school leaving age, has made him into an intellectual. The intellectual grasp of reality is an essential feature of the Western civilisation. Attitudes to life and life's problems shaped by intellectually-orientated and science-based education are deeply ingrained in the character or personality structure of Westerners from all walks of life. But they badly need the deeper outlook that springs only from the cultivation of the human psyche's higher aspirations which seem to have been deadened or put to sleep by the materialistic philosophy that seems to be a by-product of this scientific age. A sizeable proportion of scientists seems to believe that the human intelligence is a mere consequence of evolutionary changes in matter and that it is only an episode in the history of this unconscious and basically mechanical universe. Most people seem to be so fascinated by the material progress that advanced technology has bestowed on them that their philosophy of life has become, either consciously or unconsciously, materialistic as well. The perilous consequences for the quality of human life are only just becoming obvious and recognised, as the lack of a generally-accepted and respected code of ethics or moral behaviour in individual, communal and international life brings about crisis situations one after another.

A small proportion of people, particularly among the young, is seeking escape from the seemingly perilous cul-de-sac of our rational civilisation by dropping out. But that, of course, is no escape at all, unless suicide can be considered a remedy for an illness. There is, of course, one feature in dropping out that underlines what we were saying earlier. It turns, in its peculiar and sickly way, in the right direction, seeking satisfaction for the irrational longings of the human personality that have been neglected by our technological civilisation. And so we find, among drop-outs, followers of all kinds of watered-down, vague and twisted mystical trends, whether of the Zen-Buddhist, Hindu or witchcraft variety, but also, of course, we find the use—and mainly abuse—of the so-called "consciousness-expanding" drugs. The tendency that all the followers of these trends have in common is the desire to escape from the challenge to live up to the intellectual achievements of our culture, and to train themselves to live to its standards while struggling at the same time to satisfy and develop those constituents of their personality that have so far been neglected because the Western mind has allowed itself to be fasci. ıted by the quick succession of breath-taking scientific discoveries and the resulting technological successes.

But it requires no very deep thought to realize that the answer to our world's troubles lies not in throwing away our achievements and their originator, the intellect, nor in exchanging it for something else (like uncritical followers of Eastern gurus do), but in using the trained intellect in proper ways whereby it is capable of creating positive values, and in doing everything possible to help the neglected qualities of the human personality to catch up with the intellect in their development.

Some scientists are, of course, aware of the problem and concern themselves with the philosophical and ethical implications of scientific discoveries and their use. They can see the interrelatedness of science and human values, but it is not enough to deal with this problem purely intellectually. Here science must go or must allow man to go a step further in order to make new discoveries of a higher order than hitherto. For if there is a spiritual reality beyond the grasp of the intellect, surely it must be possible to reach it by methods congenial to those used by scientific research. It is not appropriate for the modern scientifically-trained mind to ignore this dimension and to leave it to be dealt with exclusively by exotic cults or mediaeval religious practices which are based on faith and which promise full results and proofs only after death.

Here again the Indian tradition points to a direction in which to search. Science was originally a Latin word for knowledge. It is significant that the Sanskṛt word for it is "*veda*", which is the name given to the bulk of literature that comprises the Indian religious and spiritual experience. And although it contains all the popular and theological as well as mystical-philosophical elements as do other religions like Christianity, in its highest form this experience claims to be the pure and direct knowledge of the ultimate reality, just as our science is the pure and direct knowledge of those bits of reality accessible to its methods of research. This is why Indian texts sometimes use terms like "science of religion", "Divine science" or "science of Yoga", Yoga being the tool or method of research whereby the final knowledge, the last goal of scientific endeavour, is to be achieved.

This claim is certainly then a challenge to the inquiring Western mind that it cannot ignore, at least in the long run. While testing the achievement of the Eastern mind, particularly as enabled by the uncommitted Yoga approach, it can retain its scientific method and critical analysis and proceed with this new field of inquiry both in scientific laboratories and in the laboratory of the human mind. The latter of course implies the experimenter's use and application of the Yoga method on a personal basis, not only by the study of its results on other subjects. Any success in this would also be a personal gain for the experimenter in terms of a new personal outlook and knowledge on a higher and deeper level of experience. It would bring a new sense of fulfilment into his life, and his work would have an immense significance for human life in general. It would represent a major break-through which could never be brought about by the current method of acquiring ever new data and creating ever new theories about reality.

Meanwhile, before any real scientific onslaught on the merits of the Yoga method begins, the popular Yoga movement in the West is likely to continue growing, perhaps bringing disappointment to some (its satisfactions do not come with the push-button efficiency of technological gadgets), but bringing personal satisfaction, some broadening of horizons and some assistance in life's tasks and problems to those who venture on its course and persist. Clearly, it is the standing task of those who, as a result of their academic specialisation, have some expert grasp of the subject to contribute as best they can to the quality of the popularisation of Yoga by introducing into it some of the necessary critical alertness and discrimination.

# BIBLIOGRAPHY


Abendländische Therapie und östliche Weisheit. Ein Tagesbericht. Ed. by Prof. W. Ritter, Stuttgart 1968.

*Addison, J.T.* : Life Beyond Death, London 1933.

*Allen, E.L.* : Existentialism from Within, London 1953.

*Aurobindo Ghosh* : On the Vedas, Pondicherry 1956.

„ „ The Life Divine, Pondicherry 1872.

*Basham, A.L.* : The Wonder that was India, London 1971 (first 1954).

*Bernard, Theos* : Hatha Yoga, London 1969 (first 1950).

*Blackham, H.J.* : Six Existentialist Thinkers, London 1956.

*Bose, A.C.* : Hymns from the Vedas, London 1966.

*Boss, M.* : A Psychiatrist Discovers India, London 1965.

*Brunton, P.* : A Search in Secret India, London 1934.

„ : The Hidden Teaching Beyond Yoga, London 1941.

„ : The Wisdom of the Overself, London (without date).

*Byles, M.B.* : Journey into Burmese Silence, London 1962.

*Choudhari, R.* : Vrātyas in Ancient India, Varanasi 1964.

*Conze, E.* : Buddhism. Its Essence and Development, Oxford 1961.

„ : Buddhist Thought in India, London 1962.

*Dasgupta, S.* : A History of Indian Philosophy I-V, Cambridge 1922-55.

„ : A study of Patañjali, Calcutta 1920.

„ : Yoga as Philosophy and Religion, London 1924.

„ : Yoga Philosophy in relation to Other Systems of Indian Thought, Calcutta 1930.

*Dayal, Har* : The Bodhisattva Doctrine in Buddhist Sanskrit Literature, London 1932 (repr. Delhi 1970).

*Desen, W.* : The Tragic Finale. An Essay on the Philosophy of Jean-Paul Sartre, Cambridge 1954.

*Deussen, Paul*: Allgemeine Geschichte der Philosophie I-II, Leipzig 1920 (first 1894-1917).

*Deussen, Paul* : Das System des Vedānta, Leipzig 1923 (first 1883), English edition Chicago 1912.

*Deutsch, E.* : Advaita Vedānta : A Philosophical Reconstruction, Honolulu 1969.

*Deutsch, E, van Buitenen, J.A.B.* : A Source Book of Advaita Vedānta, Honolulu 1971.

*Dhammasuddhi, Sobhana* : Insight Meditation, 2nd ed. London 1968.

*Dutt, Guru* : Existentialism and Indian Thought, 3rd ed. Bangalore 1960.

*Eliade, M.* : Yoga, Immortality and Freedom, 2nd ed. London 1969 (first 1958, French original 1954).

*Enomiya-Lassalle, Hugo M.* : Zen—Weg zur Erleuchtung, Wien 1960.

„ : Zen-Buddhismus, Köln 1966.

*Feuerstein, G.—Miller, J.* : A Reappraisal of Yoga, London 1971.

Forms and Techniques of Altruistic and Spiritual Growth. A Symposium. Ed. by P.A. Sorokim. Boston 1954.

*Garbe, R.* : Sāmkhya und Yoga, Strassburg 1898.

„ : Die Sāmkhya-Philosophie. 2. Aufl. Leipzig 1917.

*Glasenapp, H.v.* : Die Religionen Indiens, Stuttgart 1943.

„ : Der Stufenweg zum Göttlichen, Baden Baden 1948.

*Gonda, J.* : Die Religionen Indiens I. Veda and älterer Hinduismus, Stuttgart 1960.

*Griswold, H.D.* : The Religion of the Ṛg Veda, London, 1923.

*Grønbech, V.* : "Primitive Religionen" in 'Handbuch der Religionsgeschichte" 1, pp. 11-54 (1971; Danish in 1969).

*Hacker, P.* : Die Schule Shankaras, Wiesbaden 1951.

*Hariharānanda Āranya* : Yoga Philosophy of Patañjali, Calcutta

*Hauer, J.W.* : Die Anfange der Yoga-Praxis im alten Indien, Stuttgart 1922.

„ : Das Vrātya. Untersuchungen über die nicht-brahmanische Religion Alt-Indiens, Stuttgart 1927.

„ : Der Yoga. Ein indischer Weg zum Selbst, Stuttgart 1958.

*Hecker, H.* : Das buddhistische Nirvana. Hamburg 1971.

*Heinmann, F.H.*: Existentialism and the Modern Predicament. 2nd ed. London 1954.

*Herbert, J.* : Yoga, Christianisme et Civilisation, Lyon 1951.

*Hillebrandt, A.* : Vedische Mythologie, Breslau 1891-1902.

*Hohenberger, A.* : Rāmānuja. Ein Philosoph indischer Göttermystik, Bonn 1960.

*Iyengar, B.K.S.* : Light on Yoga, London 1965.

*Jacobs, H.* : Western Psychotherapy and Hindu Sadhana, London 1961.

„ : Indische Weisheit und westliche Psychotherapie, München 1965.

*Johanson, R.* : The Psychology of Nirvana, London 1969.

*Johnston, E.H.* : Early Sāṃkhya, London 1937.

*Keith, A.B.* : Religion and Philosophy of the Vedas and the Upanishads. Harvard Uni. Press 1925, repr. Delhi 1970.

„ : The Sāṃkhya System, Strassburg 1896.

*Kumar, Saroj* : Towards a Systematic Study of Vedānta, Calcutta 1931.

*Lamotte, E* : Histoire du Buddhisme Indien, Louvain 1958—.

*Larsen, G.J.* : Classical Sāṃkhya, Delhi 1969.

*Lea, F.A.* : A Defence of Philosophy, London 1962.

*Lehmann, E.* : "Die Religion der primitiven Völker" in "Kultur der Gegenwart", Teil I, Abt. III, 1, pp. 8-27 (1906).

*Lemaitre, S.* : Ramakrishna et la vitalité de l'hindouisme, Paris 1959.

*Macdonell, A.A.* : Vedic Mythology, Stuttgart 1897.

*Mahasi Sayadaw* : Practical Insight Meditation, Kandy 1971.

„ : The Progress of Insight, Kandy 1965.

*Marshall, A.* : Hunting the Guru in India, London 1963.

*McGovern, W.M.* : A Manual of Buddhist Philosophy, London 1923.

*Mouni Sadhu* : In Days of Great Peace, London 1952.

*Müller, M.* : Vedic Hymns (SBE 32), Oxford 1891.

„ : Three Lectures on Vedānta, London 1894.

„ : Ramakrishna, His Life and Sayings, London 1923 (first 1896).

*Mukerji, G.J.* and *Spiegelhoff, W.* : Yoga und unsere Medizin, Stuttgart 1963.

*Nyanaponika Thera* : The Heart of Buddhist Meditation, London 1962.

*Oldenberg, H.* : Die Religion des Veda, Darmstadt 1970 (first 1894).

" : Die Weltanschauung der Brāhmaṇatexte, Göttingen 1919.

" : Die Lehre der Upanishaden und die Anfänge des Buddhismus, 2nd ed, Göttingen 1923.

*Passmore, J.* : A Hundred Years of Philosophy, London 1966 first 1957).

*Radhakrishnan, S.* : Indian Philosophy I-II-London 1951 (first 1923).

" : The Principal Upanishads, London 1953.

" : The Brahma Sūtra. The Philosophy of Life, London 1960.

*Radhakrishnan, S.* and *Moore, C.A.* (ed.) : A Source Book in Indian Philosophy, Princeton 1957.

*Rahurkar, V.G.* : The Seers of the Ṛg Veda, Poona 1964.

*Raju, P.T.* : Introduction to Comparative Philosophy, Lincoln 1962.

*Arasteh, A. Reza* : Final Integration in the Adult Personality, Leyden 1965.

*Rolland, R.* : The Life of Ramakrishna, Calcutta 1965 (first 1929).

*Rolland, R.* : The Life of Vivekananda, Almora 1944 (first 1929).

*Rrytz Johansen J.* : "Definitionen und Wissenschaften von den Religionen" in "Handbuch der Religionsgeschichte" I, pp. 1-10 (1974, Danish in 1969).

*Sastri, K.* : An Introduction to Advaita Philosophy, Calcutta 1926.

*Sen Gupta, A.*: The Evolution of the Samkhya School of Thought, Patna 1959.

*Sharma H.D.* : Contributions to the History of Brahmanical Asceticism, Poona 1959.

*Shattock, E.H.* : An Experiment in Mindfulness, London 1958.

Sri Aurobindo in Selbstzeugnissen und Bilddokumenten. Dargestellt von O. Wolff, Rowohlt 1967.

Śri Maharshi. A short Life Sketch, 4th ed. Tiruvannamalai 1963.

*Srinivasa Chari S.M.* : Advaita and Viśiṣṭādvaita, London 1961.

*Srinivasa R.S.* : Contemporary Indian Philosophy, Delhi 1965.

*Srinivasa, G.* : The Existentialist Concepts and the Hindu Philosophical Systems, Allahabad 1967.

*Suzuki, D.T.* : Outlines of Mahayana Buddhism, London 1907.

*Taimni, I.K.* : The Science of Yoga, Adyar 1965.

*Tawney, C.H.* : "A Modern Hindu Saint" in "Imperial and Quarterly Review", January 1896.

The Collected Works of Ramana Maharshi. Ed. and annotated by A. Osborne, London 1959.

The Integral Philosophy of Sri Aurobindo. A Commemorative Symposium. Ed. by H. Chaudhuri and F. Spiegelberg, London 1960.

*Thomas, E.J.* : The History of Buddhist Thought, London 1933.

*Vajirañāṇa Mahāthera* : Buddhist Meditation in Theory and Practice, Colombo 1962.

*Veltheim-Ostrau, Hans-Hasso von* : Tagebücher aus Indien, Hamburg 1955.

*Venkatarama Iyer, M.K.* : Advaita Vedānta, London 1964.

*Wach, J.* : The Comparative Study of Religions, New York 1958.

*Warder A.K.* : Indian Buddhism, Delhi 1970.

*Welbon, G.D.* : The Buddhist Nirvāṇa and its Western Interpreters, Chicago-London 1968.

*Werner, K.* : "Religious Practice and Yoga in the Time of the Vedas, Upaniṣads and Early Buddhism" in "Annals of the Bhandarkar Oriental Research Institute", vol. LVI, pp. 179-194, Poona 1975.

*Wilson, Colin* : Introduction to the New Existentialism, London 1966.

*Woods, J.H.* : The Yoga System of Patañjali, Harvard 1914, repr. Delhi 1966.

*Woodward, F.L.* : Some Sayings of the Buddha, London 1960 (repr.).

*Yesudian, S.—Haich, E.* : Sport und Yoga, Thielle 1949.
Yoga and Health, London 1953.

*Zimmer, H.* : Der Weg zum Selbst : Leben und Lehre des indischen Heiligen Shri Ramana Maharshi aus Tiruvannamalai. Mit einem Vorwort hrsg. von C.G. Jung. Neuausgabe Zürich 1954.

# INDEX

# ERRATA

| Page | line | WRONG | CORRECT |
|---|---|---|---|
| 4 | 3 from bottom | in our century | in modern time |
| 24 | 12 | In the last two decades | Since the middle of the last century |
| 25 | 4 from bottom | ākāśa | *ākāśa* |
| 36 | 4-3 from bottom | promoted in recent times | promoted since early 20[th] century |
| 38 | 10 | game( *līlā*) | game (*līlā*) |
| 41 | 12 from bottom | *arūpa vacara* | *arūpāvacara* |
| 41 | 10 from bottom | *rūpa vacara* | *rūpāvacara* |
| 41 | 6 from bottom | *kāma vacara* | *kāmāvacara* |
| 42 | 13 from bottom | *kāma vacara* | *kāmāvacara* |
| 42 | 12 from bottom | *rūpa vacara* | *rūpāvacara* |
| 45 | 8 from bottom | 3,110,400 | 311,040.000 |
| 49 | note 1. | Rrytz | Prytz |
| 60 | 16-15 from bottom | gained, Thus | gained. Thus |
| 89 | note 1. | | See supplement given below |
| 94 | 18 from bottom | lonelinessis | loneliness is |
| 110 | 4 from bottom | explanation | exclamation |
| 124 | 18 | moralbehaviour | moral behaviour |
| 130 | note 1, line | *piè ce* | *pièce* |
| 136 | § 4. | *Prānayāma* | *Prāṇayāma* |
| 144 | § 4. | *mukṣatva* | *Mumukṣutva* |

| | | | |
|---|---|---|---|
| 155 | 3 | sannyāsi | *saṅnyāsi* |
| 155 | 5 | *saṅnyāsi* | *samādhi* |
| 156 | note 1. line 4 | A Modern Hindu | "A Modern Hindu |
| 157 | 10 | samādhi | *samādhi* |
| 157 | 7 from bottom | last century | 19th century |
| 158 | 10-11 | last century | 19th century |
| 158 | 13 | this century | 20th century |
| 160 | note 1. line 9 | quality. | quality: |
| 164 | 10 | Śankara | Śaṅkara |
| 165 | 19 from bottom | this century | 20th century |
| 165 | 6 from bottom | this century | 20th century |
| 170 | 4 | last two or three decades | during the 2nd half of the 20th century |

P. 89, note 1. At the end of the note please add the following:

A number of research works and comprehensive works on Mahāyāna Buddhism have been published since the first edition of this book. One of the most comprehensive ones is:

Williams, Paul, *Mahāyana Buddhism: The Doctrinal Foundations*, Routledge, London, 1989; 2nd ed. Routledge, London & New York, 2009.